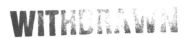

Contemporary Endodontics

Guest Editor

FREDERIC BARNETT, DMD

DENTAL CLINICS OF NORTH AMERICA

www.dental.theclinics.com

April 2010 • Volume 54 • Number 2

SAUNDERS an imprint of ELSEVIER, Inc.

W.B. SAUNDERS COMPANY
A Division of Elsevier Inc.

1600 John F. Kennedy Boulevard ● Suite 1800 ● Philadelphia, Pennsylvania 19103-2899

http://www.dental.theclinics.com

DENTAL CLINICS OF NORTH AMERICA Volume 54, Number 2
April 2010 ISSN 0011-8532, ISBN-13: 978-1-4377-1811-9

Editor: John Vassallo; j.vassallo@elsevier.com
Developmental Editor: Donald Mumford

Dental Clinics of North America (ISSN 0011-8532) is published quarterly by Elsevier Inc., 360 Park Avenue South, New York, NY 10010-1710. Months of issue are January, April, July, and October. Business and Editorial Offices: 1600 John F. Kennedy Boulevard, Suite 1800, Philadelphia, PA 19103-2899. Periodicals postage paid at New York, NY and additional mailing offices. Subscription prices are $224.00 per year (domestic individuals), $382.00 per year (domestic institutions), $108.00 per year (domestic students/residents), $266.00 per year (Canadian individuals), $481.00 per year (Canadian institutions), $321.00 per year (international individuals), $481.00 per year (international institutions), and $162.00 per year (international and Canadian students/residents. International air speed delivery is included in all *Clinics* subscription prices. All prices are subject to change without notice. **POSTMASTER:** Send address changes to *Dental Clinics of North America*, Elsevier Health Sciences Division, Subscription Customer Service, 3251 Riverport Lane, Maryland Heights, MO 63043. **Customer Service (orders, claims, online, change of address): Elsevier Health Sciences Division, Subscription Customer Service, 3251 Riverport Lane, Maryland Heights, MO 63043. Tel: 1-800-654-2452 (U.S. and Canada). Fax: 314-447-8029. E-mail: journalscustomerservice-usa@elsevier.com (for print support); journalsonlinesupport-usa@elsevier.com (for online support).**

Reprints. For copies of 100 or more, of articles in this publication, please contact the Commercial Reprints Department, Elsevier Inc., 360 Park Avenue South, New York, NY 10010-1710. Tel.: 212-633-3812; Fax: 212-462-1935; E-mail: reprints@elsevier.com.

The *Dental Clinics of North America* is covered in *MEDLINE/PubMed (Index Medicus), Current Contents/Clinical Medicine, ISI/BIOMED* and *Clinahl*.

Printed in the United States of America.

Contributors

GUEST EDITOR

FREDERIC BARNETT, DMD
Chairman and Program Director, IB Bender Division of Endodontics, Albert Einstein Medical Center, Philadelphia, Pennsylvania

AUTHORS

W.R. BOWLES, DDS, MS, PhD
Associate Professor, Department of Restorative Sciences, University of Minnesota School of Dentistry, Minneapolis, Minnesota

GARY B. CARR, DDS
Diplomate, American Board of Endodontics; Founder and Director, Pacific Endodontic Research Foundation, Private Practice, San Diego, California; Clinical Professor, Department of Endodontics at University of Texas Health Science Center, San Antonio, Texas; Clinical Professor, Department of Endodontics, University of Southern California, Los Angeles, California

DAVID CLARK, DDS
Private Practice, Tacoma, Washington

ELISABETTA COTTI, DDS, MS
Professor and Chairman, Department of Conservative Dentistry and Endodontics, School of Dentistry, University of Cagliari, Cagliari, Italy

MELISSA DRUM, DDS, MS
Assistant Professor, Department of Endodontics, The Ohio State University College of Dentistry, Columbus, Ohio

P.D. ELEAZER, DDS, MS
Professor and Chairman, Department of Endodontics and Pulp Biology, University of Alabama at Birmingham, Birmingham, Alabama

YUAN GAO, DDS, PhD
Assistant Professor of State Key Laboratory of Oral Diseases, West China College & Hospital of Stomatology, Sichuan University, Chengdu, China

MARKUS HAAPASALO, DDS, PhD
Professor, Head of the Division of Endodontics, Department of Oral Biological & Medical Sciences, UBC Faculty of Dentistry, The University of British Columbia, Vancouver, British Columbia, Canada

JOHN KHADEMI, DDS, MS
Private Practice, Durango, Colorado

CARLOS A.F. MURGEL, DDS, PhD
President of the Brazilian Micro Dentistry Association, Brazil; Visiting Faculty and Researcher at Pacific Endodontic Research Foundation, San Diego, California; Professor of Microendodontics, Department of Endodontics and Microdentistry, Campinas Dental Association, Rua Francisco Bueno de Lacerda; Private Practice, Rua Dr Sampaio Peixoto, Campinas, SP, Cep, Brazil

STEPHEN P. NIEMCZYK, DMD
Director, Endodontic Microsurgery, Harvard School of Dental Medicine, Post Graduate Endodontic Program, Boston, Massachusetts; Director, Endodontic Microsurgery, Albert Einstein Medical Center, Dental Division, Post Graduate Endodontic Program, Philadelphia, Pennsylvania; Consultant, Graduate Endodontic Program, National Naval Medical Center, Bethesda, Maryland; Consultant, United States Army Endodontic Program, Fort Gordon, Georgia; Private Practice, Drexel Hill, Pennsylvania

JOHN M. NUSSTEIN, DDS, MS
Associate Professor and Chair, Division of Endodontics, The Ohio State University College of Dentistry, Columbus, Ohio

CORNELIS H. PAMEIJER, DMD, MScD, DSc, PhD
Professor Emeritus, Department of Reconstructive Sciences, University of Connecticut Health Center, Farmington; DLC International, Simsbury, Connecticut

WEI QIAN, DDS, PhD
Resident, Graduate Endodontics Program, Faculty of Dentistry, The University of British Columbia, Vancouver, British Columbia, Canada

AL READER, DDS, MS
Professor Emeritus and Program Director, Advanced Endodontics, Division of Endodontics, The Ohio State University College of Dentistry, Columbus, Ohio

MARGA REE, DDS, MSc
Private Practice, Purmerend, The Netherlands

RICHARD S. SCHWARTZ, DDS
Clinical Assistant Professor, Graduate Endodontics, University of Texas Health Science Center at San Antonio, San Antonio, Texas

YA SHEN, DDS, PhD
Clinical Assistant Professor, Division of Endodontics, Department of Oral Biological & Medical Sciences, UBC Faculty of Dentistry, The University of British Columbia, Vancouver, British Columbia, Canada

MARTIN TROPE, DMD
Clinical Professor, University of Pennsylvania, Philadelphia, Pennsylvania; Professor Emeritus, University of North Carolina School of Dentistry, Chapel Hill, North Carolina

OSVALDO ZMENER, DDS, Dr Odont
Head Professor, Post Graduate Program for Specialized Endodontics, Faculty of Medical Sciences, School of Dentistry, University of El Salvador, Buenos Aires, Argentina

Contents

> In the last 15 years, there has been an explosion of new technologies, instruments, and materials for nonsurgical and surgical endodontics. These developments have improved the precision with which endodontics is performed. The most important revolution has been the introduction and widespread adoption of the operating microscope (OM). Its introduction into dentistry, particularly in endodontics, has revolutionized how endodontics is practiced worldwide. This article provides basic concepts on how an OM is implemented and used in clinical endodontic practice and also gives an overview of its clinical and surgical applications.

> Imaging is an important clinical aid for the diagnosis of endodontic bone lesions. Traditional radiology performs more accurately than ever. Computed tomography has been used for the last 20 years with important implications in the management of lesions in bone. Among the newest systems, digital volume tomography is becoming a new standard and real-time echotomography is gaining an interesting space in the diagnostic field of endodontics. These techniques offer some advantages for the increased safety and the amount of detailed information they can provide.

> Attaining local anesthesia for the treatment of teeth diagnosed with irreversible pulpitis ("hot" tooth) can be a challenge. This article looks at the strategies a dentist can use to help achieve adequate pulpal anesthesia for the patient, thereby eliminating or reducing treatment pain.

> During patient treatment, the clinician needs to consider the operator needs, the restoration needs, and the tooth needs. This article discusses molar access and failures of endodontically treated teeth that occur not because of chronic or acute apical lesions but because of structural compromises to the teeth that ultimately render them useless. The authors believe that the current models of endodontic treatment do not lead to

long-term success, and that the traditional approach to endodontic access is fundamentally flawed. This article introduces a set of criteria that will guide the clinician in treatment decisions to maintain optimal functionality of the tooth and help in deciding whether the treatment prognosis is poor and alternatives should be considered.

The following case studies provide insight into the integration of the principles set forward in the preceding article. Each case is evaluated first on the endorestorative principles that form the basis of the modern endo-endorestorative–prosthodontic continuum. Case 1 is provided by Dr Clark, and cases 2 to 6 are provided by Dr Khademi.

The success of endodontic treatment depends on the eradication of microbes from the root-canal system and prevention of reinfection. The root canal is shaped with hand and rotary instruments under constant irrigation to remove the inflamed and necrotic tissue, microbes/biofilms, and other debris from the root-canal space. Irrigants have traditionally been delivered into the root-canal space using syringes and metal needles of different size and tip design. Clinical experience and research have shown, however, that this classic approach typically results in ineffective irrigation. Many of the new compounds used for irrigation have been chemically modified and several mechanical devices have been developed to improve the penetration and effectiveness of irrigation. This article summarizes the chemistry, biology, and procedures for safe and efficient irrigation and provides cutting-edge information on the most recent developments.

Traditional methods of treatment of immature root with necrotic pulp and apical periodontitis pose multiple challenges. These challenges include disinfection of the root canal with standard protocols that aggressively use endodontic files, filling the root canal with an open apex that provides no barrier for stopping the root filling material before impinging on the periodontal tissues, and the susceptibility of the teeth to fracture because of their thin roots. Disinfection using sodium hypochlorite, apical barrier formation using calcium hydroxide as well as mineral trioxide aggregate, and pulp revascularization of immature tooth with the help of blood clot and collagen-enhanced matrix has been discussed in detail in this article.

With the appearance of more in vivo and ex vivo publications, methacrylate based resin sealers are becoming more popular in endodontics. Their ease of use and favorable clinical performance offer an attractive alternative to conventional endodontics. This article reviews the development of resin-based sealers and biocompatibility tests. The many, mostly opposing views are analyzed to put what has been published thus far in perspective. A critical analysis of the facts leads to the consensus that methacrylate based resin sealers are here to stay and offer a suitable alternative to conventional endodontic treatment.

Successful endodontic treatment depends on the restorative treatment that follows. The connection between endodontic treatment and restorative dentistry is well accepted, but the best restorative approaches for endodontically treated teeth have always been somewhat controversial. A plethora of information from various sources contributes to the controversy and much of it is contradictory. With the emergence of implants in mainstream dentistry, there has been more emphasis on long-term outcomes and on evaluating the "restorability" of teeth prior to endodontic treatment. The long-term viability of endodontically treated teeth is no longer a "given" in the implant era. In consequence, some teeth that might have received endodontic treatment in the past are now extracted and replaced with implant-supported prostheses if they are marginally restorable or it makes more sense in the overall treatment plan. As it is not possible to review here all the literature on the restoration of endodontically treated teeth, this article focuses primarily on current concepts based on the literature from the past 10 years or so, and provides treatment guidelines based on that research.

While endodontic microsurgery has been making tremendous strides in the past 20 years, there are still basic concepts that are confusing or frustrating for the novice and experienced surgeon alike. These issues, such as microscope positioning and the relationship with the surgeon's ergonomics and line of sight to the surgical field, making use of natural hand movements and positions, are addressed in this article. Other topics include major flap designs and guidelines for their implementation, effective hemostasis using materials with less tissue toxicity, root end preparation techniques and guidelines, site-determined choice of root end filling material, and placement and finishing tips for Mineral Trioxide Aggregate.

Dental professionals are often faced with challenges when formulating a treatment plan for patients presenting with a compromised tooth. A common dilemma involves the decision between tooth retention using endodontic treatment with crown restoration, and extraction and an implant-borne restoration. In this article the authors evaluate the 2 treatment modes, and observe that because outcomes are similar with both treatments, decisions should be based on the patient's informed decision concerning restorability, costs associated with the procedures, esthetics, potential adverse outcomes, and ethical factors.

RELATED INTEREST

Oral and Maxillofacial Surgery Clinics of North America May 2009 (Vol. 21, No. 2)
Current Controversies in Maxillofacial Trauma
Daniel M. Laskin, DDS, MS, and A. Omar Abubaker, DMD, PhD, *Guest Editors*

THE CLINICS ARE NOW AVAILABLE ONLINE!

Access your subscription at:
www.theclinics.com

Preface

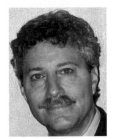

Frederic Barnett, DMD
Guest Editor

The focus of this issue is on contemporary clinical endodontics. As there have been several fundamental changes in the specialty of endodontics over the last years, the purpose of this issue is to inform our dental colleagues about these changes. Each article offers realistic information, most of which can be put to immediate use in clinical practice. As such, the clinician will benefit directly from the up-to-date information in this issue.

The authors include leading national and international authorities in their field. A broad and diversified range of topics has been chosen for this issue. The topics range from advanced techniques for detecting bone lesions, anesthesia for the hot tooth, contemporary access designs, root filling with resin materials, access restoration, and endodontic surgery. Additionally, an article on the endodontic–implant decision tree has been included.

I would like to thank the authors for generously contributing their knowledge, passion, and expertise to this issue. It is my hope that reading this issue of *Dental Clinics of North America* will enhance the level of skill and understanding of endodontics for our dental colleagues.

Frederic Barnett, DMD
IB Bender Division of Endodontics
Albert Einstein Medical Center
Philadelphia, PA, USA

E-mail address:
barnettf@einstein.edu

Dent Clin N Am 54 (2010) xi
doi:10.1016/j.cden.2010.01.004
0011-8532/10/$ – see front matter © 2010 Elsevier Inc. All rights reserved.

dental.theclinics.com

The Use of the Operating Microscope in Endodontics

Gary B. Carr, DDS[a,b,c,d,]*, Carlos A.F. Murgel, DDS, PhD[a,e,f,g]

KEYWORDS

• Operating microscope • Magnification • Endodontics

Endodontists have frequently boasted that they can do much of their work blindfolded simply because there is "nothing to see." The truth is that there is a great deal to see with the right tools.[1]

In the last 15 years, for nonsurgical and surgical endodontics, there has been an explosion in the development of new technologies, instruments, and materials. These developments have improved the precision with which endodontics is performed. These advances have enabled clinicians to complete procedures that were once considered impossible or that could be performed only by talented or lucky clinicians. The most important revolution has been the introduction and widespread adoption of the operating microscope (OM).

OMs have been used for decades in other medical disciplines: ophthalmology, neurosurgery, reconstructive surgery, otorhinolaryngology, and vascular surgery. Its introduction into dentistry in the last 15 years, particularly in endodontics, has revolutionized how endodontics is practiced worldwide.

Until recently, endodontic therapy was performed using tactile sensitivity, and the only way to see inside the root canal system was to take a radiograph. Performing

[a] Pacific Endodontic Research Foundation, 6235 Lusk Boulevard, San Diego, CA 92121, USA
[b] Department of Endodontics, University of Texas Health Science Center, 7703 Floyd Curl Drive, San Antonio, TX 78229, USA
[c] Department of Endodontics, University of Southern California, 925 West 34th Street, Los Angeles, CA 90089-0641, USA
[d] Private Practice, San Diego, CA 92121, USA
[e] Brazilian Micro Dentistry Association, Brazil
[f] Department of Endodontics and Microdentistry, Campinas Dental Association, Rua Francisco Bueno de Lacerda 30, Pq. Italia, Campinas - SP 13030-900, Brazil
[g] Private Practice, Rua Dr Sampaio Peixoto, 206, Campinas, SP, Cep 13024-420, Brazil
* Corresponding author. Pacific Endodontic Research Foundation, 6235 Lusk Boulevard, San Diego, CA 92121.
E-mail address: gary@tdo4endo.com

Dent Clin N Am 54 (2010) 191–214
doi:10.1016/j.cden.2010.01.002
0011-8532/10/$ – see front matter © 2010 Published by Elsevier Inc.

dental.theclinics.com

endodontic therapy entailed "working blind," that is, most of the effort was taken using only tactile skills with minimum visual information available. Before the OM, the presence of a problem (a ledge, a perforation, a blockage, a broken instrument) was only "felt," and the clinical management of the problem was never predictable and depended on happenstance. Most endodontic procedures occurred in a visual void, which placed a premium on the doctor's tactile dexterity, mental imaging, and perseverance.

The OM has changed both nonsurgical and surgical endodontics. In nonsurgical endodontics, every challenge existing in the straight portion of the root canal system, even if located in the most apical part, can be easily seen and competently managed under the OM. In surgical endodontics, it is possible to carefully examine the apical segment of the root end and perform an apical resection of the root without an exaggerated bevel, thereby making class I cavity preparations along the longitudinal axis of the root easy to perform.

This article provides basic information on how an OM is used in clinical endodontic practice and an overview of its clinical and surgical applications.

ON THE RELATIVE SIZE OF THINGS

It is difficult, even for a scientist, to have an intuitive understanding of size. Specifically, a dentist must have an accurate understanding of the relationship between the gross dimensions involved in restorative procedures and the dimensions of deleterious elements that cause restoration failure, such as bacteria, open margins, and imperfection in restorative materials. A filling or a crown may appear well placed, but if bacteria can leak through the junction between the tooth and the restorative material, then treatment is compromised.

A brief review of relative size may be helpful. Cell size is measured in microns (millionths of a meter, μm), and a single bacterial cell is about 1 μm in diameter. One cubic inch of bacteria can hold about a billion cells. A typical human (eukaryotic) cell is 25 μm in diameter, so an average cell can hold more than 10,000 bacteria. By comparison, viruses are so small that thousands can fit within a single bacterial cell. Simple calculations show that 1 in^3 can contain millions of billions of viruses. These calculations do not end there. For example, the size of macromolecules (eg, bacterial toxins) is measured in nanometers, or one-billionth of a meter (**Fig. 1**).

Some of these bacterial toxins are so potent that even nanogram quantities can cause serious complications and even death. Clearly, dentists are at a severe disadvantage in their attempts to replace natural tooth structure with artificial materials that do not leak, in view of the virtually invisible microbiologic threats to restoration integrity.[2]

THE LIMITS OF HUMAN VISION

Webster defines resolution as the ability of an optical system to make clear and distinguishable 2 separate entities. Although clinicians have routinely strived to create bacteria-free seals, the resolving power of the unaided human eye is only 0.2 mm. Most people who view 2 points closer than 0.2 mm will see only 1 point. For example, **Fig. 2** shows an image of a dollar bill. The lines making up George Washington's face are 0.2mm apart. If the bill is held close enough, one can probably just barely make out the separation between these lines. If they were any closer together, you would not be able to discern that they were separate lines. The square boxes behind Washington's head are 0.1 mm apart and not discernible as separate boxes by most people. The

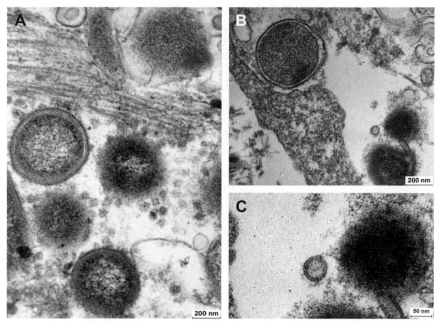

Fig. 1. (*A*) Bacterial blebbing from gram-negative biofilm bacteria. (*B*) Membrane-enclosed bleb. (*C*) Higher magnification of bleb. (*From* Carr GB, Schwartz RS, Schaudinn C, et al. Ultrastructural examination of failed molar retreatment with secondary apical periodontitis: an examination of endodontic biofilms in an endodontic retreatment failure. J Endod 2009;35(9):1303–9; with permission.) (Pacific Endodontic Research Foundation.)

boxes are beyond the resolving power of the unaided human eye. For the sake of comparison, it would take about 100 bacteria to span that square. Clinically, most dental practitioners will not be able to see an open margin smaller than 0.2 mm. The film thickness of most crown and bridge cements is 25 μm (0.025 mm), well beyond the resolving power of the naked eye.

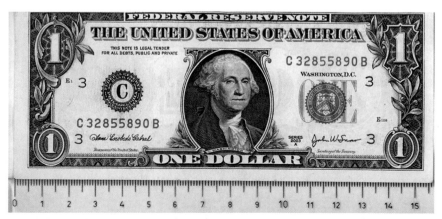

Fig. 2. A dollar bill without magnification. Note that the lines that make George Washington's face cannot be seen in detail.

Optical aids (eg, loupes, OMs, surgical headlamps, fiberoptic handpiece lights) can improve resolution by many orders of magnitude. For example, a common OM can raise the resolving limit from 0.2 mm to 0.006 mm (6 μm), a dramatic improvement. **Fig. 3** shows the improvement in resolution obtained by the standard OM used in dentistry today. A clinical example is that at the highest power a restoration margin opening of only 0.006 mm is essentially sealed and this is beyond the common cement thickness film used in restorative dentistry.

WHY ENHANCED VISION IS NECESSARY IN DENTISTRY

Any device that enhances or improves a clinician's resolving power is extremely beneficial in producing precision dentistry. Restorative dentists, periodontists, and endodontists routinely perform procedures requiring resolution well beyond the 0.2-mm limit of human sight. Crown margins, scaling procedures, incisions, root canal location, caries removal, furcation and perforation repair, postplacement or removal, and bone- and soft-tissue grafting procedures are only a few of the procedures that demand tolerances well beyond the 0.2-mm limit.

OPTICAL PRINCIPLES

Because all clinicians must construct 3-dimensional structures in a patient's mouth, stereopsis, or 3-dimensional perception, is critical to achieving precision dentistry. Dentists appreciate that the human mouth is a small space to operate in, especially considering the size of the available instruments (eg, burs, handpieces) and the comparatively large size of the operator's hands. Attempts have been made to use the magnifying endoscopes used in artroscopic procedures, but these devices require viewing on a 2-dimensional (2D) monitor, and the limitations of working in 2D space are too restrictive to be useful.

Several elements are important for consideration in improving clinical visualization. Included are factors such as

Stereopsis
Magnification range
Depth of field
Resolving power
Working distance
Spherical and chromatic distortion (ie, aberration)
Ergonomics
Eyestrain
Head and neck fatigue
Cost.

Dentists can increase their resolving ability without using any supplemental device by simply moving closer to the object of observation. This movement is accomplished in dentistry by raising the patient up in the dental chair to be closer to the operator or by the operator bending down to be closer to the patient.[2] This method is limited, however, by the eye's ability to refocus at the diminished distance.

Most people cannot refocus at distances closer than 10 to 12 cm. Furthermore, as the eye-subject distance (ie, focal length) decreases, the eyes must converge, creating eyestrain. As one ages, the ability to focus at closer distances is compromised. This phenomenon is called presbyopia and is caused by the lens of the eye losing flexibility with age. The eye (lens) becomes unable to accommodate and

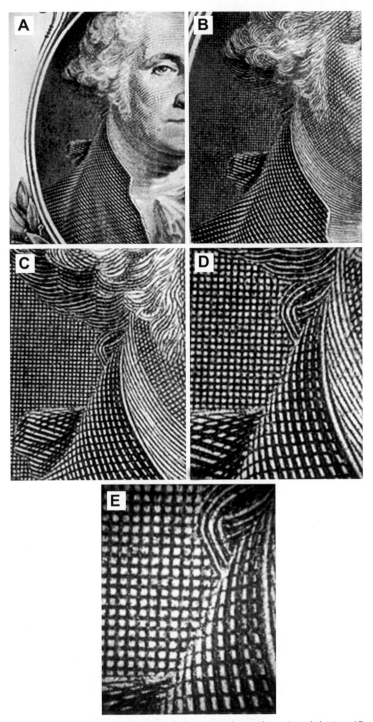

Fig. 3. Different magnifications of a dollar bill as seen through an OM. (*A*) Magnification ×3. (*B*) Magnification ×5. (*C*) Magnification ×8. (*D*) Magnification ×10. (*E*) Magnification ×18.

produce clear images of near objects. The nearest point that the eye can accurately focus on exceeds ideal working distance.[3]

As the focal distance decreases, depth of field decreases. Considering the problem of the uncomfortable proximity of the practitioner's face to the patient, moving closer to the patient is not a satisfactory solution for increasing a clinician's resolution. Alternatively, image size and resolving power can be increased by using lenses for magnification, with no need for the position of the object or the operator to change.

LOUPES

Magnifying loupes were developed to address the problem of proximity, decreased depth of field, and eyestrain occasioned by moving closer to the subject. (Depth of field is the ability of the lens system to focus on objects that are near or far without having to change the loupe position. As magnification increases, depth of field decreases. Also, the smaller the field of view, the shallower the depth of field. For a loupe of magnification ×2, the depth of field is approximately 5 in [12.5 cm]; for a loupe of magnification ×3.25, it is 2 in [6 cm]; and for a loupe of magnification ×4.5, it is 1 in [2.5 cm].)

Loupes are classified by the optical method by which they produce magnification. There are 3 types of binocular magnifying loupes: (1) a diopter, flat-plane, single-lens loupe, (2) a surgical telescope with a Galilean system configuration (2-lens system), and (3) a surgical telescope with a Keplerian system configuration (prism-roof design that folds the path of light).

The diopter system relies on a simple magnifying lens. The degree of magnification is usually measured in diopters. One diopter (D) means that a ray of light that would be focused at infinity would now be focused at 1 meter (100 cm or 40 in). A lens with 2 D designation would focus light at 50 cm (19 in); a 5 D lens would focus light at 20 cm (8 in). Confusion occurs when a diopter single-lens magnifying system is described as 5 D. This designation does not mean ×5 power (ie, 5 times the image size). Rather, it signifies that the focusing distance between the eye and the object is 20 cm (<8 in), with an increased image size of approximate magnification ×2 (2 times actual size). The only advantage of the diopter system is that it is the most inexpensive system. But it is less desirable because the plastic lenses that it uses are not always optically correct. Furthermore, the increased image size depends on being closer to the viewed object, which can compromise posture and create stresses and abnormalities in the musculoskeletal system.[3]

The surgical telescope of either the Galilean or the Keplerian design produces an enlarged viewing image with a multiple-lens system that is positioned at a working distance between 11 and 20 in (28–51 cm). The most used and suggested working distance is between 11 and 15 in (28–38 cm).

The Galilean system provides a magnification range from ×2 to ×4.5 and is a small, light, and compact system (**Fig. 4**).

The prism loupes (Keplarian system) use refractive prisms and are actually telescopes with complicated light paths, which provide magnifications up to ×6 (**Fig. 5**).

Both systems produce superior magnification and correct spherical and chromatic aberrations, have excellent depth of field, and are capable of increased focal length (30–45 cm), thereby reducing eyestrain and head and neck fatigue. These loupes offer significant advantages over simple magnification eyeglasses.

The disadvantage of loupes is that the practical maximum magnification is only about ×4.5. Loupes with higher magnification are available, but they are heavy and unwieldy,

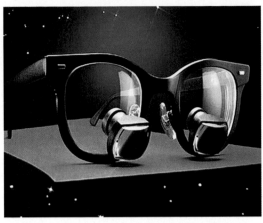

Fig. 4. An example of a Galilean system. (*Courtesy of* Designs for Visions, Inc, Ronkonkoma, NY, USA.)

with a limited field of view. Using computerized techniques, some manufacturers can provide magnifications from ×2.5 to ×6 with an expanded field. Nevertheless, such loupes require a constrained physical posture and cannot be worn for long periods of time without producing significant head, neck, and back strain.

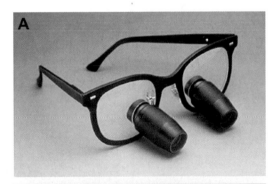

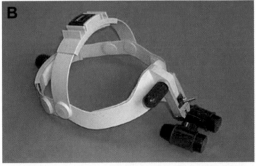

Fig. 5. An example of a Galilean system. (*A*) Prism loupes. These loupes have sophisticated optics, which rely on internal prisms to bend the light. (*Courtesy of* Designs for Visions, Inc, Ronkonkoma, NY, USA.) (*B*) Headset and prism loupes. (*Courtesy of* Carl Zeiss, Inc, Germany.)

THE PROBLEM OF LIGHT

By increasing light levels, one can increase apparent resolution (the ability to distinguish 2 objects close to each other as separate and distinct). Light intensity is determined by the inverse square law, which states that the amount of light received from a source is inversely proportional to the square of the distance. For example, if the distance between the source of light and the subject is decreased by half, the amount of light at the subject increases 4 times. Based on the law, therefore, most standard dental operatory lights are too far away to provide the adequate light levels required for many dental procedures.

Surgical headlamps have a much shorter working distance (13 in or 35 cm) and use fiberoptic cables to transmit light, thereby reducing heat to minimal levels. Another advantage is that the fiberoptic cable is attached to the doctor's headband so that any head movement moves the light accordingly. Surgical headlamps can increase light levels up to 4 times that of conventional dental lights (**Fig. 6**).

THE OM IN ENDODONTICS

Apotheker introduced the dental OM in 1981.[1] The first OM was poorly configured and ergonomically difficult to use. It was capable of only 1 magnification ($\times$8), was positioned on a floor stand and poorly balanced, had only straight binoculars, and had a fixed focal length of 250 mm. This OM used angled illumination instead of confocal illumination. It did not gain wide acceptance, and the manufacturer ceased

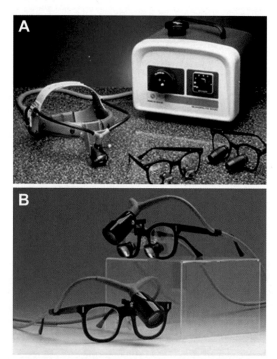

Fig. 6. Surgical headlight and loupes. Together, these devices can greatly increase a clinician's resolution. (*Courtesy of* Designs for Visions, Inc, Ronkonkoma, NY, USA.)

manufacturing it shortly after its introduction.[4] Its market failure was more a function of its poor ergonomic design than its optical properties, which were actually good.

Howard Selden[5] was the first endodontist to publish an article on the use of the OM in endodontics. He discussed its use in the conventional treatment of a tooth, not in surgical endodontics.

In 1999, Gary Carr[6,7] introduced an OM that had Galilean optics and that was ergonomically configured for dentistry, with several advantages that allowed for easy use of the scope for nearly all endodontic and restorative procedures. This OM had a magnification changer that allowed for 5 discrete magnifications (magnification ×3.5–×30), had a stable mounting on either the wall or ceiling, had angled binoculars allowing for sit-down dentistry, and was configured with adapters for an assistant's scope and video or 35-mm cameras (**Fig. 7**).

It used a confocal illumination module so that the light path was in the same optical path as the visual path, and this arrangement gave far superior illumination than the angled light path of the earlier scope. This OM gained rapid acceptance within the endodontic community, and is now the instrument of choice not only for endodontics but for periodontics and restorative dentistry as well. The optical principles of the dental OM are seen in **Fig. 8**.

The efficient use of the OM requires advanced training. Many endodontic procedures are performed at magnification ×10 to ×15, and some require a magnification as high as ×30. Operating comfortably at these magnifications requires accommodation to new skills that were not taught until recently in dental schools. Among other things, working at these higher-power magnifications brings the clinician into the realm where even slight hand movements are disruptive, and physiologic hand tremor is a problem.

In 1995, the American Association of Endodontists formally recommended to the Commission on Dental Accreditation of the American Dental Association that microscopy training be included in the new Accreditation Standards for Advanced Specialty Education Programs in Endodontics. At the commission's meeting in January 1996, the proposal was agreed on, and in January 1997, the new standards, making microscopy training mandatory, became effective.[8]

EFFICIENT USE OF AN OM IN ENDODONTICS

Although the OM is now recognized as a powerful adjunct in endodontics, it has not been adopted universally by all endodontists. It is seen by many endodontists as simply another tool and not as a way of practice that defines how an endodontist works. Although cost is frequently cited as the major impediment, in truth, it is not

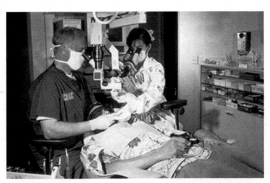

Fig. 7. Today's OM allows the doctor and the assistant to ergonomically view the same field. This OM is fitted with a 3CCD (charge coupled device) video camera and an assistant scope.

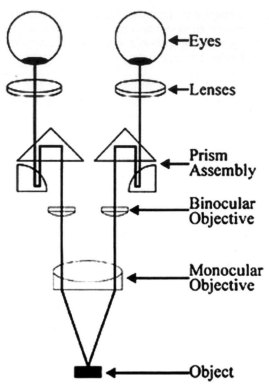

Fig. 8. Galilean optics. Parallel optics enables the observer to focus at infinity, relieving eyestrain.

cost but a failure to understand and implement the positional and ergonomic skills necessary to effectively use an OM. This failure has restricted its universal use in all endodontic cases.

The occasional or intermittent use of an OM on a patient results in the inefficient use of a clinician's time. It represents a disruption in the flow of treatment of the patient, which can only negatively affect the final result. Clinicians who practice this way seldom realize the full advantage of a microscopic approach and never develop the visual and ergonomic skills necessary to operate at the highest level.

The skillful use of an OM entails its use for the entire procedure from start to finish. Working in such a way depends on refinement of ergonomic and visual skills to a high level.

THE LAWS OF ERGONOMICS

An understanding of efficient workflow using an OM entails knowledge of the basics of ergonomic motion. Ergonomic motion is divided into 5 classes of motion:

Class I motion: moving only the fingers (**Fig. 9**)
Class II motion: moving only the fingers and wrists (**Fig. 10**)
Class III motion: movement originating from the elbow (**Fig. 11**)
Class IV motion: movement originating from the shoulder (**Fig. 12**)
Class V motion: movement that involves twisting or bending at the waist.

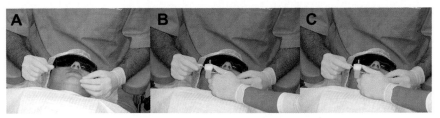

Fig. 9. (*A*) Fingers waiting for the file. (*B*) File placed in between fingers. (*C*) Fingers capturing file.

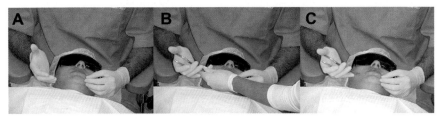

Fig. 10. (*A*) Hand waiting for the instrument. (*B*) Fingers and wrist movement receiving the instrument. (*C*) Fingers movement receiving the instrument.

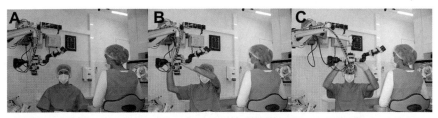

Fig. 11. (*A*) Elbow rested at the stool support. (*B*) Supported elbow rotation and instrument apprehension. (*C*) Supported elbow rotation to working position.

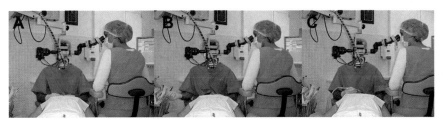

Fig. 12. (*A*) Professional at the neutral position. (*B*) Shoulders, arms, elbows, and hands moving to reach the OM. (*C*) OM moved to the ideal position without rotational movement of the waist.

No clinical example of the Class V motion movement is shown because this movement is the most prejudicial of all (unfortunately, this is the most common movement used by dentists and dental assistants with or without the OM).

POSITIONING THE OM

The introduction of the OM in a dental office requires significant forethought, planning, and an understanding of the required ergonomic skills necessary to use the OM efficiently. Proper positioning for the clinician, patient, and assistant is absolutely necessary. Most problems in using an OM in a clinical setting are related to either positioning errors or lack of ergonomic skills in the clinician. If proper ergonomic guidelines are followed, it is possible to work with the OM in complete comfort with little or no muscle tension.

In chronologic order, the preparation of the OM involves the following maneuvers:

Operator positioning
Rough positioning of the patient
Positioning of the OM and focusing
Adjustment of the interpupillary distance
Fine positioning of the patient
Parfocal adjustment
Fine focus adjustment
Assistant scope adjustment.

OPERATOR POSITIONING

The correct operator position for nearly all endodontic procedures is directly behind the patient, at the 11- or 12-o'clock position. Positions other than the 11- or 12-o'clock position (eg, 9-o'clock position) may seem more comfortable when first learning to use an OM, but as greater skills are acquired, changing to other positions rarely serves any purpose. Clinicians who constantly change their positions around the scope are extremely inefficient in their procedures.

The operator should adjust the seating position so that the hips are 90° to the floor, the knees are 90° to the hips, and the forearms are 90° to the upper arms.[9] The operator's forearms should lie comfortably on the armrest of the operator's chair, and feet should be placed flat on the floor. The back should be in a neutral position, erect and perpendicular to the floor, with the natural lordosis of the back being supported by the lumbar support of the chair. The eyepiece is inclined so that the head and neck are held at an angle that can be comfortably sustained. This position is maintained regardless of the arch or quadrant being worked on. The patient is moved to accommodate this position. After the patient has been positioned correctly, the armrests of the doctor's and assistant's chairs are adjusted so that the hands can be comfortably placed at the level of the patient's mouth. The trapezius, sternocleidomastoid, and erector spinae muscles of the neck and back are completely at rest in this position.

Once the ideal position is established, the operator places the OM on one of the lower magnifications to locate the working area in its proper angle of orientation. The image is focused and stepped up to higher magnifications if desired.[10]

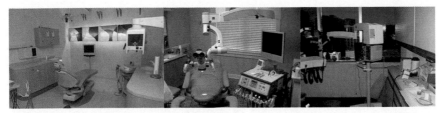

Fig. 13. Examples of traditional operatory designs with large side cabinets, sinks, and so forth. A design such as this makes efficient OM use problematic.

OPERATORY DESIGN PRINCIPLES FOR USING OM

The OM was originally introduced into standard dental operatories that have been designed in the conventional way, with outdated ergonomic concepts using the traditional operatory side cabinets, dual sinks, over-the-patient delivery systems, and so forth. This historical design turned out to be extremely inefficient because of the ergonomic constraints imposed by the way the OM is actually used in endodontic procedures. There is an ergonomic flow to using an OM efficiently, and careful operatory design is critical in enabling this flow. One of the main reasons clinicians struggle with using the OM for all procedures is that the ergonomic design of the operatory prohibits it. Clinicians who attempt to use the OM for all procedures but do not have appropriate ergonomic designs to their operatories experience significant frustrations (**Fig. 13**).

The organizing design principle using the OM in the dental operatory should revolve around an ergonomic principle called circle of influence (**Fig. 14**). The principle posits that all instruments and equipment needed for a procedure are within reach of either the clinician or the assistant, requiring no more than a class IV motion, and that most endodontic procedures are performed with class I or class II motions only (**Fig. 15**). The principle assumes that the most ergonomic way to work is to perform all procedures under the OM, including the diagnostic examination, oral cancer screening, anesthesia, and rubber dam placement.

Therefore, the circle of influence design principle places the OM at the center of the operatory design, and all the ergonomic movements necessary to work with this technology are centered within those circles. Simplicity and efficiency are the guiding principles of this innovative design. This innovative concept allows for the constant evolution of the operatory design while maintaining its ergonomic parameters and permitting the incorporation of new technologies as they become available.

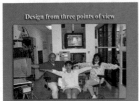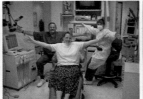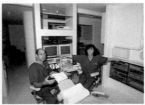

Fig. 14. The circle of influence design takes into consideration the 3 participants of the dental team: doctor, assistant, and patient. Maximum ergonomics, efficiency, and comfort for all members are achieved with this office design.

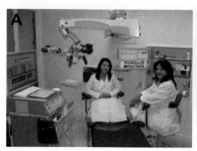
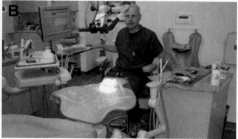

Fig. 15. The circle of influence principle can be implemented into private practice (*A*) and in the academic environment (*B*) (Einstein Medical Center, Philadelphia, PA, USA).

The design has been improved to make it even simpler to implement and less expensive by adopting off-shelf solutions from IKEA (PA, USA). This design is extremely valuable, especially because of its availability and ease of setup. In a few hours, one can construct an ideal OM operatory back wall using all the circle of influence design principles for a fraction of the cost of a traditional operatory with custom cabinets (**Fig. 16**).

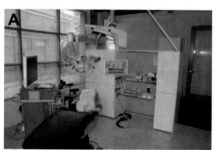
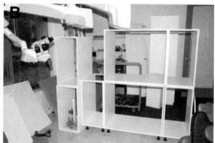
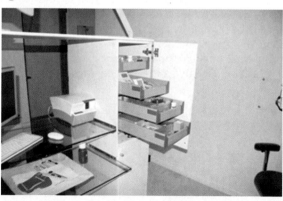
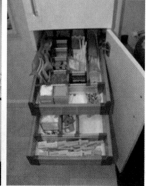

Fig. 16. (*A*) The circle of influence design concept using different IKEA cabinets. Note how spacious and clean this design is, in contrast to traditional ones. The key elements here are rear-mounted or ceiling mounted OM, cart, back wall, assistant table, stool with arm support, computer integration, and rotational chair. (*B*) Ease of construction using modular design principles. (*C*) Efficient IKEA delivery cabinets.

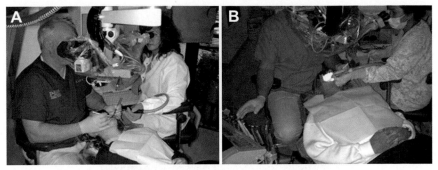

Fig. 17. (*A*) Team work development: doctor and assistant working erect and muscularly relaxed. (*B*) Adjustable cart allowing access to all instruments, using only a class III motion.

KEY ELEMENTS OF THE NEW DESIGN

This new design assumes a teamwork approach to the delivery of endodontic care. The doctor and assistant are placed at the scope in upright and comfortable positions (**Fig. 17**A). The scope is positioned so that the doctor and the assistant are muscularly at rest through all treatment phases (see **Fig. 17**A). This configuration places some constraints on the design of the back wall and on the cart systems used. Computers, scanners, digital radiographs, and monitors are ergonomically placed according to the circle of influence principle and are easily reached by either the doctor or the assistant with only class III motions (**Fig. 17**B). The cart must be easily movable and adjustable and at the correct height to be ergonomically positioned (see **Fig. 17**B).

The dental chair is freely rotatable with the doctor's legs, so that the patient, not the OM, is moved when a field of view needs to be changed. Patient movement, and not OM movement, is a paradigm shift in understanding how to use an OM efficiently. The small rotational movement of the dental chair should be done using the practitioner's legs and not hands (**Fig. 18**). This simple principle can change the way one practices. In this position, the patient faces the ceiling, and the practitioner works around at the 11-o'clock position for nearly every procedure. Doctor and assistant stools with arm support are critical (**Fig. 19**). Because fine motor skills are necessary to work under

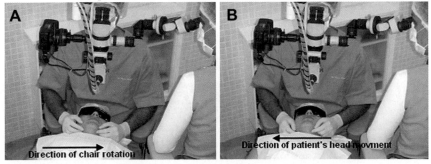

Fig. 18. (*A*) Small movement of the chair to the left (note that patient's head is tilted a little to the left). (*B*) If necessary, the patient's head is moved slightly to the right to compensate chair movement (note that the OM was not touched at any time).

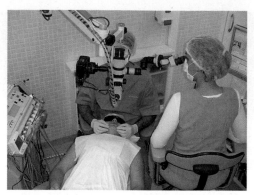

Fig. 19. Elbow support for doctor and assistant is mandatory to allow the necessary fine motor skills under constant magnification and muscular comfort throughout the day.

constant magnification, it is mandatory that both members have adequate elbow and arm support. Without either support, fine motor skills with either hand become more problematic for the practitioner and for the dental assistant (**Fig. 20**).

THE OM AND CLINICAL PROCEDURES

The efficient use of an OM for all clinical procedures requires not only ergonomic sophistication but also special clinical skills that are not required in nonmicroscopic endodontics. When one tries to use conventional concepts with magnification, frustration and inefficiency are the usual results (**Fig. 21**). Specifically, in microendodontics, the use of specialized micromirrors vastly improves efficiency and capability (**Fig. 22**). The skills needed to manipulate much smaller mirrors at higher magnification are easily acquired by dentists, but not without some effort. The use of smaller mirrors results in the mirror being placed further away from its usual location, and even minor hand movements can make such use frustrating for the novice (**Fig. 23**). Proper ergonomic form and a well-trained assistant can mitigate some of this frustration, but it takes practice and repetition to master the skills required (**Fig. 24**).

Removing canal or pulp chamber obstructions is also greatly facilitated by the use of an OM. Even obstructions such as separated instruments deep within canals can be addressed, given the proper training and level of persistence. Examining fractures,

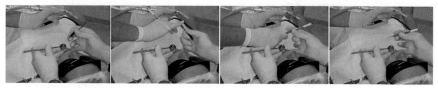

Fig. 20. A simple exchange of instruments demands fine motor skills once the doctor and assistant are going to ideally use class I, II, and III movements (note how the doctor's hands does not leave the reference point at patient's cheek).

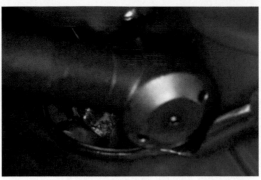

Fig. 21. Image with intermediate magnification (×6) of access on tooth No.15. Nothing is seen besides the high-speed head and parts of the tooth. Such image when using the OM, causes frustration and introduces inefficiency and significant clinical impairment.

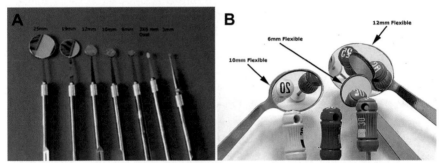

Fig. 22. (*A*) A selection of flexible mirrors in different sizes and shapes. (*B*) Detail of highly reflective mirrors with flexible and flat shafts. (*Courtesy of* EIE2, San Diego, USA.)

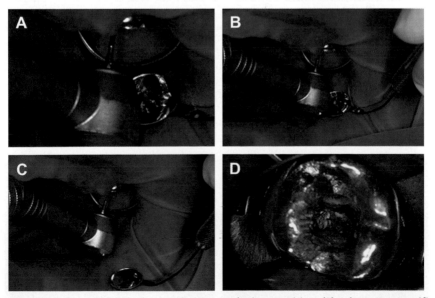

Fig. 23. (*A*) Inadequate level of magnification and mirror position. (*B*) Adequate magnification to position mirror. (*C*) Adequate mirror position. Notice the flex of the mirror staff. (*D*) Adequate magnification level with clear view of the operatory field.

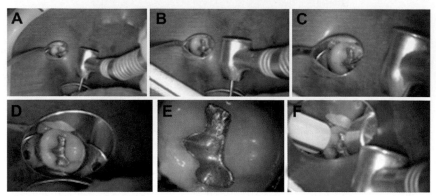

Fig. 24. (*A*) The use of smaller mirrors positioned further away. Adequate level of magnification and mirror position. (*B–E*) Higher magnifications of occlusal surface. (*F*) Clear view of occlusal surface ready to initiate clinical work with high speed and suction well position.

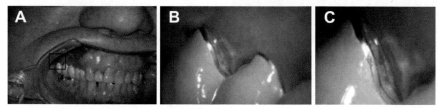

Fig. 25. Clinical diagnosis of prosthetic margins. (*A*) Low magnification of crown on tooth No. 2. (*B*) Intermediary magnification of crown margin. (*C*) High magnification of crown margin.

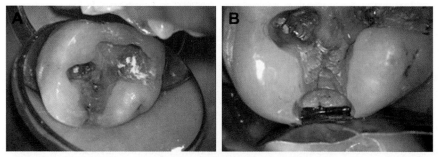

Fig. 26. Clinical diagnosis of cracks. (*A*) Intermediary magnification of occlusal surface of tooth No. 2. (*B*) Higher magnification showing cracks on distal area.

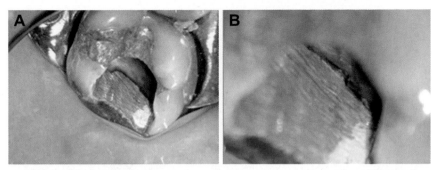

Fig. 27. Clinical diagnosis of caries. (A) Intermediary magnification of occlusal surface on tooth No. 14. (B) Higher magnification showing gross microleakage and an open margin on cervical area.

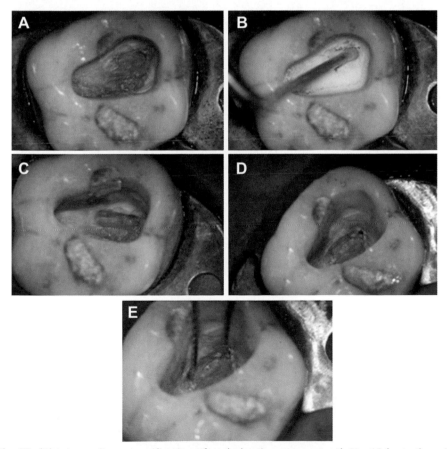

Fig. 28. (A) Intermediary magnification of endodontic access on tooth No. 15 (note there is no sign of canals). (B) Dentin smear resulted from ultrasonic instrumentation (Pearl diamond, EIE2 Excellence in Endodontics, GBC Innovations, Inc, San Diego, CA, USA) of pulp floor. (C) Groove produced after ultrasonic usage. (D) Mesiobuccal (MB) and second MB (MB2) canals located after ultrasonic usage. (E) Files inserted on MB and MB2 canals.

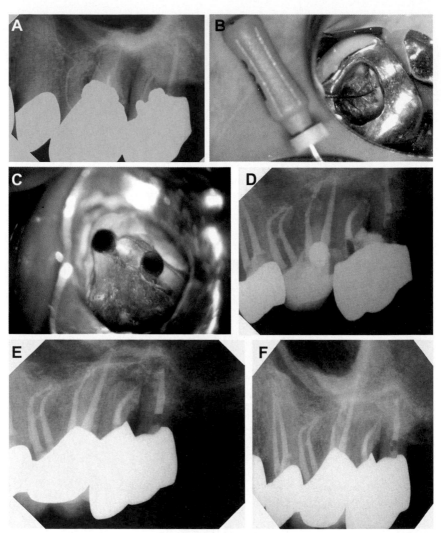

Fig. 29. (*A*) Preoperative radiograph of teeth Nos. 13, 14 and 15 showing inadequate previous root canal treatment (teeth 14 and 15) with incomplete shaping and obturation of the root canal system. (*B*) Intermediary magnification of 06 file at MB2. (*C*) Higher magnification showing MB and MB2, cleaned and shaped. (*D*) Immediately postoperation. (*E, F*) Long-term recall.

crown margins, cement layers, subgingival defects, and caries extension are all enhanced by a microscopic approach.

To discuss the uses of the OM in endodontics is beyond the scope of this article, but several examples of its use serve to illustrate its permanent place in endodontics.

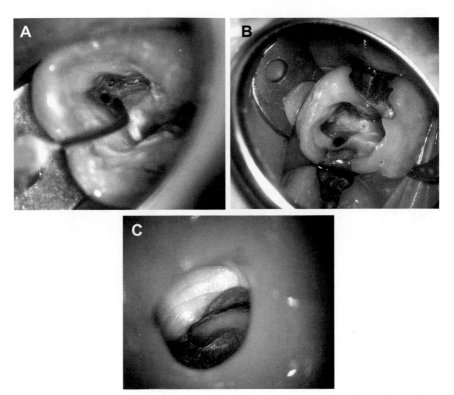

Fig. 30. Intermediate magnification of tooth No. 2 with an extra distal lingual canal (white spot dehydrated with air).

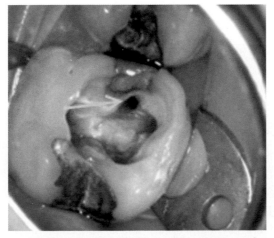

Fig. 31. Intermediate magnification of tooth No. 3 with an MB2 canal way under the mesial ridge.

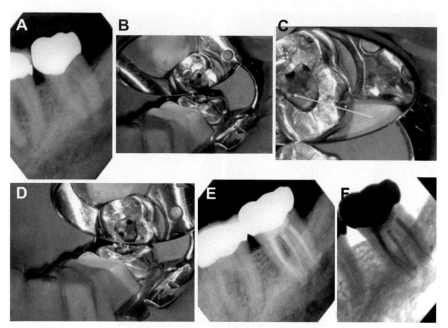

Fig. 32. (*A*) Preoperative radiograph of tooth No. 18 showing the presence of chronic apical periodontitis, but no sign of aberrant anatomy. (*B*) Low magnification of mesial canals, cleaned and shaped. (*C*) Higher magnification showing extra mesial lingual canal (*arrow*). (*D*) Low magnification of mesial lingual canal, cleaned and shaped. (*E*) Immediate postoperative radiograph, (*F*) Immediate postoperative inverted radiograph.

Clinical Diagnosis

In endodontics, clinical diagnosis has a greater need for enhanced vision. With the advent of implant dentistry, a more accurate diagnosis is necessary to select only viable and long-lasting teeth that will withstand the test of time (**Figs. 25–27**).

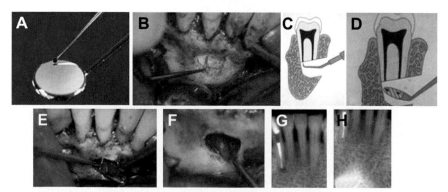

Fig. 33. (*A*) Regular and retro mirror comparison. (*B*) Apical exploration after root resection. (*C, D*) Microsurgery technique. (*E*) Ultrasonic retro preparation. (*F*) Retro preparation filled. (*G*) Immediately postoperation. (*H*) Long-term recall.

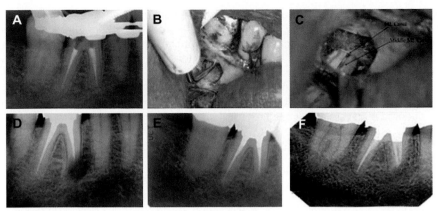

Fig. 34. (*A*) Before operation. (*B*) Ultrasonic root preparation with moderated bevel, (*C*) Micromirror view of retropreparation, (*D*) Immediately postoperation. (*E*) 5-year recall. (*F*) 10-year recall.

Locating Canals

Locating canals is perhaps the most obvious use of the OM in endodontics. Calcified canals (**Fig. 28**), missed canals (**Fig. 29**), aberrant canals (**Figs. 30–32**), dilacerated canals, and canals blocked by restorative materials are all addressed easily by the skillful use of an OM.

Operators quickly learn the visual skills necessary to distinguish dentin from calcified pulp, relying on changes in color, translucency, and refractive indexes to identify remnants of pulpal tissues. Such searches have historically resulted in perforations or gross destruction of tooth structure, but with the advent of the OM, such misadventures are uncommon.

Surgical Endodontics

Modern endodontic surgical procedures demand a microscopic approach. Use of the smaller retro mirrors allow for a more moderated bevel of the root resection and permit a coaxial ultrasonic preparation into the root (**Figs. 33** and **34**).[6]

Surgical soft-tissue management is also greatly enhanced by a microscopic approach, leading to faster healing, less traumatic soft-tissue management, and the advent of microsurgical suturing techniques that minimize trauma and lead to rapid, primary intention wound healing (**Fig. 35**).

These are only a few of the endodontic applications of a microscopic approach, but there are others such as lateral root repairs, perforation repairs, external cervical

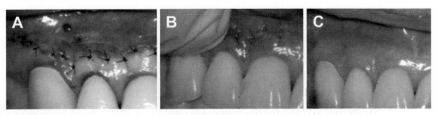

Fig. 35. (*A*) Immediately postoperation. (*B*) 48 hours postoperation. (C) 21 days postoperation. Incision scar barely visible.

invasive resorption repairs, and other resorptive repairs that also benefit from a microscopic approach. In reality, all clinical endodontic procedures should be done under constant illumination, magnification, and ergonomics. This requirement applies even for implant dentistry, which needs special attention to fine details to achieve excellence.[10]

As the OM gains widespread acceptance in endodontics, the advantages of its use in providing precision care will carry over into restorative dentistry, and it will eventually become a universal approach for all phases of dentistry.[4,10–15]

REFERENCES

1. Apotheker H. A microscope for use in dentistry. J Microsurg 1981;3(1):7–10.
2. Friedman S, Lustmann J, Shahardany V. Treatment results of apical surgery in premolar and molar teeth. J Endod 1991;17(1):30–3.
3. Weller N, Niemczyk S, Kim S. The incidence and position of the canal isthmus: part 1. The mesiobuccal root of the maxillary first molar. J Endod 1995;21(7): 380–3.
4. Carr GB. Magnification and illumination in endodontics. In: Hardin FJ, editor. Clark's clinical dentistry, vol. 4. St Louis, MO: Mosby; 1998. p. 1–14.
5. Selden HS. The role of a dental operating microscope in improved nonsurgical treatment of "calcified" canals. Oral Surg Oral Med Oral Pathol 1989;68(1):93–8.
6. Carr GB. Common errors in periradicular surgery. Endod Rep 1993;8(1):12–8.
7. Carr GB. Microscopes in endodontics. J Calif Dent Assoc 1992;20(11):55–61.
8. Selden HS. The dental-operating microscope and its slow acceptance. J Endod 2002;28(3):206–7.
9. Michaelides PL. Use of the operating microscope in dentistry. J Calif Dent Assoc 1996;24(6):45–50.
10. Sheets CG, Paquette JM. The magic of magnification. Dent Today 1998;17(12): 60–3, 65–7.
11. Worschech CC, Murgel CAF. Micro-odontologia: visão e precisão em tempo real. Londrina: Dental Press International; 2008. p. 31–81.
12. Carr GB. Endodontics at the crossroads. J Calif Dent Assoc 1996;24(12):20–6.
13. Carr GB. Ultrasonic root end preparation. Dent Clin North Am 1997;41(3):541–54.
14. Castellucci A. Magnification in endodontics: the use of the operating microscope. Pract Proced Aesthet Dent 2003;15(5):377–84.
15. Murgel CAF, Gondim E Jr, Souza Filho FJ. Microscópio Cirúrgico: a busca da excelência na Clínica Odontológica [Surgical Microscope: the search for excellence on clinical dentistry]. Rev da Assoc Paul Cir Dent 1997;51:31–5 [in Portuguese].

Advanced Techniques for Detecting Lesions in Bone

Elisabetta Cotti, DDS, MS

KEYWORDS

• Radiologic techniques • CBVT • CT • Echography
• Periapical lesions

Apical periodontitis (AP) is an infectious disease caused by bacteria (in association with viruses and fungi) residing in the root canal system (endodontium) of the affected teeth, and organized in a biofilm as a consequence of pulpal infection and necrosis.[1–3] The pathogenesis of AP is due to the initiation of a nonspecific inflammatory response and a specific immunologic reaction of the host in the periradicular tissues (cementum of the tooth, periodontal ligament, and alveolar bone) in response to the infection coming from the endodontium. The establishment of this response is considered an attempt from the body to prevent the spread of the infection deep into the bone. As the disease proceeds it causes resorption of the periapical bone and its substitution with the inflammatory tissue.[1,4,5] Clinical signs and symptoms that may be associated with the different stages of this pathologic condition are represented by soft tissue swelling, presence of a sinus tract, and pain on percussion of the tooth and on palpation of the periapical area. However, it is the presence of osteolytic lesions in the periapical/periradicular area of the maxillary bones that represents the clinical landmark of AP.[4,5]

The changes in the mineralization and structure of the periapical bone that can be seen by radiographic techniques are the major indicator of the presence of AP and the progression of its healing **(Fig. 1)**.[5,6]

From a histopathologic perspective, bone radiolucencies caused by AP may be distinguished as periapical cysts and granulomas.[7,8] Furthermore, two kinds of lesions can be identified among periapical cysts; the true cyst (a cavity completely enclosed in its epithelial lining with no direct connection to the apical portion of the root canal) and the periapical pocket cyst (a cavity lined by epithelium that forms a collar around the apex of the involved tooth and that is consequently open to the root canal).[7,8] According to the results from the most reliable studies in the recent literature, the prevalence of cysts among AP is 15% of which 9% are true cysts and 6% are pocket cysts.[9] It has

Department of Conservative Dentistry and Endodontics, School of Dentistry, University of Cagliari, Via Binaghi # 4, 09100, Cagliari, Italy
E-mail address: Cottiend@tin.it

Dent Clin N Am 54 (2010) 215–235
doi:10.1016/j.cden.2009.12.007
0011-8532/10/$ – see front matter © 2010 Elsevier Inc. All rights reserved.

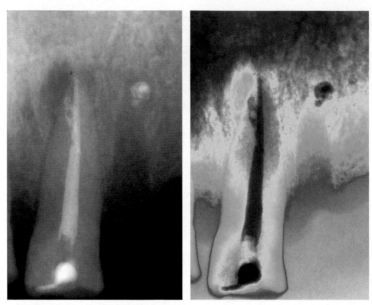

Fig. 1. Digital periapical radiographs (regular and color-coded) showing a lesion of endodontic origin.

been suggested that true cysts may sustain persistent AP, therefore it is important to make a differential diagnosis between periapical lesions using clinical and radiographic techniques,[9–12] even though histologic serial or semiserial sectioning of the whole lesion is considered the only reliable diagnostic method to date.[9] Thus, diagnostic information will directly influence the clinical decisions on the management of periapical bone lesions.

An effective imaging system is required for the following purposes:

1. Detection of all the lesions present in the maxillary bones.
2. Disclosure of the anatomic coordinates of the lesions in the three spatial dimensions for diagnostic and treatment purposes (determine shape and measures of a lesion; determine the amount of cortical bone involved; visualize the relationship of a lesion with the root tip(s) and the anatomic landmarks in the bones).
3. Orientation toward a differential diagnosis of the lesions of endodontic origin (ie, cysts vs granulomas) and of endodontic lesions versus other radiolucencies.
4. Follow-up evaluation of the outcome of the treatment.

The information may be obtained by traditional radiology (intraoral periapical radiographs and panoramic radiographs), which has the limitation of being a two-dimensional representation of three-dimensional structures.[13,14] Whenever further information is required, advanced imaging systems are needed.[6,15]

ADVANCED IMAGING TECHNIQUES

Advanced imaging systems that have become more and more helpful in the management of endodontic lesions are computed tomography (CT), cone beam volumetric tomography and ultrasound real-time echotomography. Each of these techniques has the specificity to enhance the diagnostic potential, increase the awareness of the anatomic details, make better differential diagnoses or investigate protocols.

CT and Dental CT

CT was introduced by Hunsfield[16] in the 1970s and it provides imaging of soft tissues, bone, and vessels.[17] With this technique the part of the body to be examined is divided into slices by fanning out of collimated roentgen rays. As the x-ray source rotates around the region of interest, multiple sensors detect the beam. These slices are layers consisting of volume elements known as voxels, whose height is determined by the selected thickness of the layer. The system measures the attenuation of the rays entering the anatomic structures located within these voxels from many different angles. The attenuation coefficients encountered by the rays passing through the anatomic structures (depending on the thickness and on the atomic number of the tissue elements) are detected and transformed into images. The values of attenuation coming from a linear or tangential direction are referred to as projections. The computer then reconstructs the part under observation into a series of cross sections or planes.

CT is widely used for the diagnosis of pathologic conditions in the maxillary bones.[17] Using a specific protocol of investigation and software, dental CT is a procedure that permits a metric analysis of transverse sections of the jaws in three dimensions.[18–20] In dental CT direct axial scans of the jaws are acquired using the highest possible resolution, and then secondary curved and orthoradial multiplanar tomograms are reconstructed by data computation. To avoid the influence of artifacts generated from metal restorations, the field of measurement can be positioned inferior to the occlusal plane in the jaw of interest.[20] Conventional CT, spiral CT or multislice CT can be used for dental CT. A standard protocol for dental CT in the diagnosis of pathologic conditions of the jaws should use: slice thickness of 1.5 mm, table feed of 1.0, field of view (FOV, mandible) of 120 mm, FOV (maxilla) of 100 mm, scan time of 2 seconds, voltage of 80 to 120 kV, current of 25 to 100 mA, mandible base, and hard palate as scan planes.[21] The data accumulated from the primary axial tomograms are transformed into multiplanar reconstructions using dental software. The indirect orthoradial reconstructions are calculated perpendicular to a planning line along the centreline of the jaw arch. The distance between each of the 40 to 60 cuts is 1.5 to 3.0 mm.[20] The panoramic views and cross sections of the jaws reconstructed from the axial slices make it possible to measure distances and diameters, and to determine the thickness of the osseous structures. In each single jaw examination the axial scans are displayed followed by the dental reconstructions on a 1:1 scale including the planning line, the orthoradial lines, and the dental scans, which are numbered and correlated to the orthoradial reconstructions (**Figs. 2** and **3**).

Tissue density is measured in Hounsfield units (HU) on a scale from −1000 to +3000 HU (water = 0 HU; air = −1000 HU). Bone ranges from 500 to 1300 HU (compact bone) to 100 to 240 HU (cancellous bone); soft tissue is approximately 40 HU.[20]

The major concern related to dental CT is the high radiation dose required for average examinations; in the last few years dose reduction methods have been established.[20,22] Reducing the tube current is an important step, followed by using 1.5-mm slice thickness. The spiral CTs (if used with pitch higher than 1), provide an optimum data set while drastically reducing the amount of radiation because they use continuous scanning to generate cross-sectional slices. In this examination the pitch indicates the slice thickness (in millimeters) and the rate at which the table is advanced (layers per rotation = mm/360°). By increasing the rotation speed and exposing several layers simultaneously, the exposure time and the radiation dose is reduced.

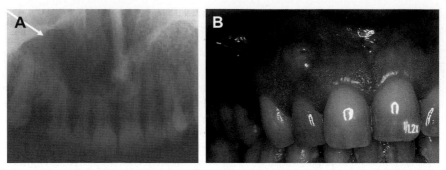

Fig. 2. (A) Details from a panoramic radiograph showing an extensive lesion (*white arrow*) of endodontic origin related to tooth no. 22. (B) Clinical photograph of the same tooth, showing the swelling in the buccal-periapical area.

An additional suggestion for dose reduction is to be specific about the area of interest for the investigation, selecting the upper or lower jaw and excluding all the occlusal scans.[20–22]

Cone Beam Volumetric Tomography

Cone beam volumetric tomography (CBVT),[20,23–25] also called digital volume tomography or cone beam CT, was developed to produce three-dimensional images of the maxillofacial region with scan time reduction and lower radiation dosage than medical-grade CT. The examination is produced using a narrow cone-shaped x-ray beam. The x-ray source and the sensor rotate synchronously between 180° and 360° around the head of the patient only once. The sensor can be either an image intensifier or a flat panel. The image intensifier can be coupled with a charged coupled device or with a complementary oxide semiconductor; the flat panel (thin film transistor) is the newest image receptor for solid large area arrays and it produces less distortion with a wider scale of contrast. The method of acquiring images in CBVT is different from medical CT. In CBVT, a single scan captures projection data in a volume and the voxels are consequently isotropic. A reconstruction algorithm then calculates the three-dimensional image of the original object. From this volume, tomographic slices from 0.125 mm thickness are displayed in 3 orthogonal planes. New slices can be also made in any direction. Three-dimensional image volume is represented in a cylinder or a sphere greater than 100 million voxels; some CBVT machines acquire larger data volumes than others. Depending on the FOV, limited CBVT can be distinguished from full CBVT. Limited CBVT creates a three-dimensional image volume in the range of 4 × 4 to 10 × 10 cm² with smaller isotropic voxels (0.125–0.2 mm), thus increasing the resolution and the accuracy of measurements. Image volumes in full CBVT range from 10 × 10 to 20 × 20 cm² (voxels = 0.2–0.4 mm). The dedicated viewer software of the CBVT system allows the clinician to examine the full volume together with the simultaneous axial, sagittal, and coronal views of the area of interest. The CBVT system obtained US Food and Drug Administration approval for dental use in the United States in 2000.[25] There are now several CBVT systems on the market. The major difference between the systems is in the detector used and in the FOV. Depending on the CBVT, the patient can be examined in a seated, standing, or supine position. CBVT uses ionizing radiation and therefore the most common concern arising is the effective radiation dose on the patient. Most of the time CBVT yields a lower effective radiation dose than traditional CT. Exposure time can be reduced

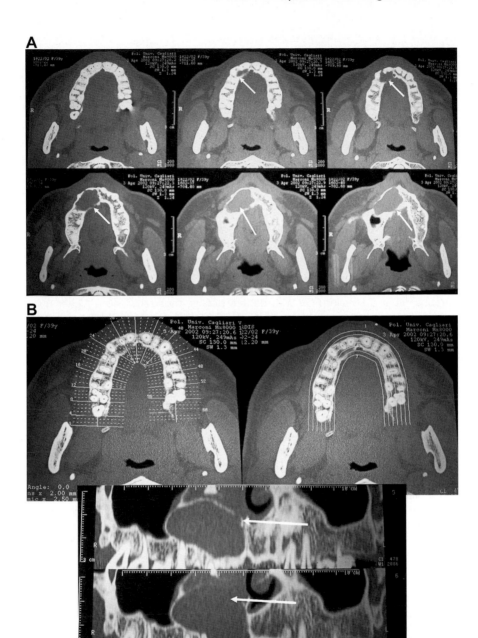

Fig. 3. (*A*) Axial scans of the previous lesion (*white arrows*) showing its extension and the involvement of the cortical plates. (*B*) Dentascan of the same lesion (*white arrows*). Involvement of the sinus is visible. (*C*) Surgical excision of the same lesion.

by using pulsating technology (making the beam-on time shorter than the scan time). The effective dose from digital panoramic radiographs ranges from 4.7 to 14.9 micro-Sieverts (µSv), and the effective dose for a full mouth series is from 33 to 84 µSv. According to the literature, not all CBVT machines deliver the same radiation dose

C

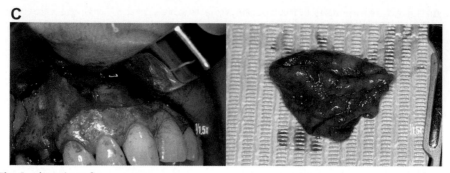

Fig. 3. (*continued*)

per examination. The amount of radiation can range from 2% to 23% of medical-grade CT and can be 4 to 42 times higher than a single panoramic radiograph (from 4.70 μSv to 134 μSv).[26–30]

To minimize the radiation dose and depending on the region of interest, the clinician might use either a smaller FOV with betters details, thus requiring a higher mA, or a bigger FOV with lower resolution, thus requiring a lower mA.[28] CBVT has been the object of numerous applications in the field of endodontics.[25,31]

Ultrasound Real-time Echotomography

This widely used imaging system is based on the reflection of ultrasound waves.[32] Ultrasound waves are generated as a consequence of the piezoelectric effect by a quartz or synthetic ceramic crystal when it is exposed to an alternating electric current of 3 to 10 MHz. Ultrasound waves oscillating at the same frequency are collimated by an acoustic lens and sent toward the area of interest in the body using a transducer, which is called an ultrasonic probe and contains a crystal.

Because the different biologic tissues in the body possess different mechanical and acoustic properties, the ultrasound waves at the interface between 2 tissues with different acoustic impedance undergo the phenomena of reflection and refraction. The echo is the part of the ultrasound wave that is reflected back from the tissue interface toward the transducer.

The transducer transforms the reflected ultrasound waves (echo) into electromagnetic waves of the same frequency, which are then transformed into images in a computer. The greater the difference in acoustic properties between 2 adjacent tissues, the higher is the intensity of the echoes originating from them. The ultrasound images seen on the computer monitor are produced by the movement of the crystal over the tissue of interest, which appear as a sequence of moving images (an average of 30 images per second). When the operator moves the probe on the examination area a change is created on the sector plane, thus producing a real-time three-dimensional image of that particular space.

If an area in a given tissue has high echo intensity, it is called hyperechoic and will appear as a white bright spot. Bone exhibits total reflection and is therefore hyperechoic. An area that has low echo intensity is called hypoechoic and appears as a darker image. An area that has no echo intensity it is called anechoic and appears very dark in the examination. Fluid-filled areas exhibit no reflection and are anechoic. Areas that contain different types of tissues show a dishomogeneous echo.

When applied to ultrasound examination, color power Doppler (CPD) flowmetry[33] allows the presence and direction of the blood flow within the tissue of interest to be observed. The intensity of the Doppler signal is represented by changes in real time on a graph (Doppler) and is also shown in the form of color spots on the gray scale image (color). Positive Doppler shifts are caused by the blood moving toward the transducer and are represented in red, whereas negative Doppler shifts are caused by blood moving in the opposite direction and are represented in blue. Power Doppler is associated with color Doppler to improve its sensitivity to low flow rates. It is based on the integrated power spectrum, and can disclose the minor vessels.[11] The use of contrast media by intravenous (IV) injections increases the echogenicity of the blood making the color power Doppler examination more sensitive.[32,33] Ultrasound imaging is a safe technique; the biologic risk is much lower than that associated with radiographs because it does not use ionizing radiations.[34–36] Potential adverse effects of ultrasound (caused by cavitation and vibration) depend on the length of time the ultrasound energy is applied; safety measures therefore limit the number of examinations.

REQUIREMENTS FOR THE DETECTION AND MANAGEMET OF ENDODONTIC LESIONS
Detection of the Lesions in the Maxillary Bone and in the Mandible

A two-dimensional digital panoramic radiograph can often be enough for the preliminary visualization of the patient's dentition and related bone pathosis, in particular, if the general condition of the teeth (caries, previous restorations) is within average. Periapical radiographs, taken in at least 2 different projections, will follow through to have a close up on selected teeth, check for the presence and extension of caries, view the condition of restorative work, and diagnose the possible lesion.[6] Treatment of the affected tooth can thus be planned.

When the overall condition of the dentition is complex because of the existence of numerous caries, restorations, and root canal treatments, then the presence of undetected periapical pathosis might be suspected and an examination that will eliminate superimposition of teeth or surrounding structures in the area of interest is required. The same consideration is valid whenever there are periapical symptoms but the lesion(s) cannot be seen with conventional two-dimensional images. CT and CBVT are then indicated.

As a result of the high resolution achieved, dental CT and then CBVT have become significantly more effective than radiographs for the detection of periapical lesions in bone.[6,37]

Velvart and colleagues[38] correlated the presence of lesions diagnosed with CT and radiographs to the actual findings in the surgical field on 50 teeth selected for endodontic surgery. The 78 lesions found during the surgical procedure were visible on the CT scans, whereas only 61 of them were seen using conventional radiographs.

Stavropoulos and Wenzel[39] used CBVT to examine experimental bone defects in pig jaws, and showed that this examination has a higher diagnostic accuracy than intraoral radiography, conventional and digital. Nakata and colleagues[40] reported a case in which, only using CBVT, they were able to detect the presence of a periapical lesion in the root of a symptomatic maxillary molar, which had not been diagnosed with intraoral and panoramic radiographs.

Lofthag-Hansen and colleagues[41] in a very comprehensive clinical work conducted at the Public Dental Health Service in Goteborg reported that CBVT provided additional information not found on periapical radiographs. In particular, in 36 patients and a total of 46 teeth analyzed, periapical lesions were diagnosed in the same 32 teeth with both examinations. However, lesions were diagnosed in 10 more teeth with the CBVT images. Among these 10, 3 undetected lesions were considerably large, crossing the alveolar bone in the bucco-palatal direction and expanding into the maxillary sinus (**Fig. 4**). Furthermore, when the lesions were correlated to individual roots, the same 53 lesions were diagnosed with both techniques and 33 more roots with lesions were seen using the volumetric tomography.

In another report 34% more lesions, particularly related to maxillary second molars or to roots in close proximity with the maxillary sinus, were seen using CBVT.[42]

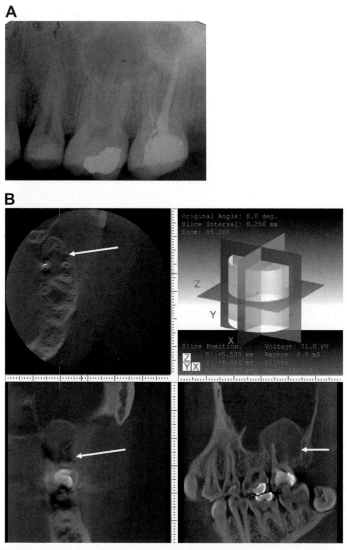

Fig. 4. (*A*) Periapical radiograph showing tooth no. 27 with what appears as a small lesion on the mesial root. (*B*) CBVT (*Courtesy of* Professor Carlo Prati [3D Accuitomo, J Morita, Mfg Corp. Kyoto, Japan].) of the same tooth no. 27 with the 3 projections: axial (*upper left*), sagittal (*lower right*), and coronal (*lower left*). In this image set, it is possible to see the huge lesion within the sinus (*arrows*), is not visible in the periapical radiograph. The volume of the examination is represented on the upper right.

Similar results were found by Estrela and his group in 2 consecutive papers. In the first study on 888 patients, they compared the accuracy of CBVT, and panoramic and periapical radiographs for the detection of AP, finding that the overall sensitivity of periapical and panoramic radiographs was 0.55 and 0.28, respectively.[43] In the second study, on 569 patients and 1014 teeth, AP was detected in 39.5% of the cases examined with the radiographs and in 60.9% of the cases screened with CBVT.[44]

Disclosure of the Anatomic Coordinates of the Lesions in 3 Spatial Dimensions

Knowing the anatomic coordinates of a lesion in 3 spatial dimensions means:

(a) To be aware of the size of a lesion at different levels in the bone and in the multiple spatial projections
(b) To understand whether and where the cortical plates are involved or perforated by the inflammatory process
(c) To determine the position and divergence of the roots within the alveolar process of the maxillary bones and their involvement in a lesion
(d) To know the proximity of a lesion/root to vital anatomic landmarks such as the mandibular canal, mental foramen, incisal canal, and maxillary sinus.

An average of 70% more clinically relevant information (of outmost importance in endodontic presurgical planning) can be gathered with CT and CBVT than with traditional radiographs (**Figs. 1–6**).[38,41–44]

CT has been advocated as a preferential imaging system when looking for details not achievable using two-dimensional examinations such as the relation of the lesions to the buccal and the lingual cortical plates, and their size. The periphery of the osteolitic lesion can be easily identified and measured on the cross-sectional reconstructions.[45] In the in vivo clinical study by Velvart and colleagues[38] mentioned earlier, all the information achieved with high-resolution CT scans made it possible to evaluate the extent of the lesions and their precise position within the bone. The oblique cuts of the same CT scans also provided the predictable identification of the mandibular canal and its relationship with the lesions and the roots. The same information was not predictably obtained in all the cases examined using radiographs. The inferior alveolar nerve and the mental foramen in relation to the apex of mandibular premolars can also be precisely located with CBVT (see **Fig. 5**).[25] The involvement of the roots/lesions with the sinus floor and their expansion into the maxillary sinus is another important concern when planning surgery, which can be overcome only using CT or CBVT (see **Fig. 2** and **3**).[42,46,47] From these examinations it was possible to show that in 76% of first molars and in 50% of second molars the sinus floor was intertwined with the roots,[42] and that it was approached by 30% of second premolar roots. The sinus was found between the buccal and the palatal root of the first molar in 25% of cases.[47] In 32% of cases, maxillary root lesions perforate the sinus, and in 30% of the cases they are separated from the sinus by 1 mm of bone or less.[42] The position and the size of the incisive foramen/canal have been determined with CT and CBVT with equal success.[25,48]

The linear and three-dimensional measurements for the anatomic structures[49,50] and volumetric measurements of osseous lesions[51] taken with CBVT are considered accurate in vitro and in vivo. The mean horizontal distance of the palatal root of the first maxillary molars from the buccal cortical plate (mean distance = 9.73 mm) has been measured by CBVT to assess surgical access.[47] Apico-marginal communications, which can be an important indication of the presence of a radicular fracture, are also more frequently detected by CBVT.[42]

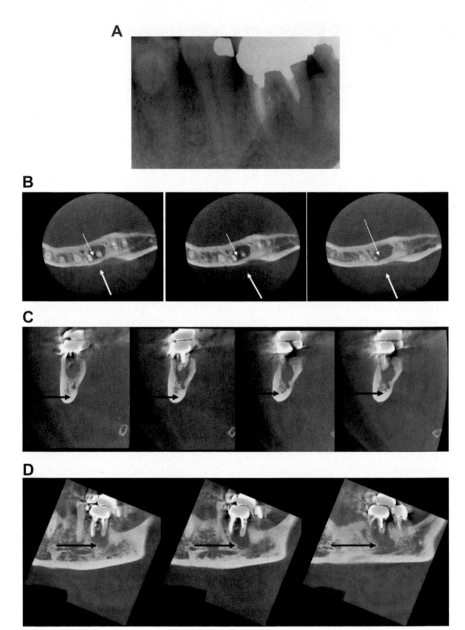

Fig. 5. (*A*) Periapical radiograph of tooth no. 36 showing a periapical lesion, a previous root canal treatment, and crown restoration. (*B*) Axial scans from CBVT (3D Accuitomo) of the same tooth in the widest portion of the lesion, showing its relationships with the cortical plates and the roots of the tooth (*arrows*). (*C*) CBVT coronal scan of the same tooth. (*D*) Sagittal scan of the same tooth. The progressive relation of the lesion with the mandibular canal is clearly visible (*arrows*).

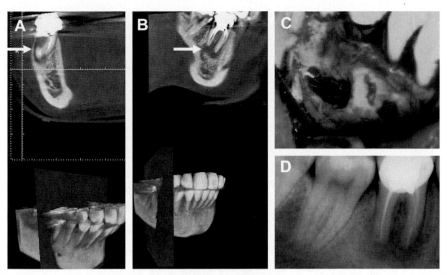

Fig. 6. (*A*) Presurgical CBVT coronal scan on tooth no. 46 (Promax, Planmeca Oy, Helsinki, Finland). It is possible to select the surgical access by assessing the slice where the cortical plate is thinner (*arrow*). (*B*) Sagittal scan showing the lesion with respect to the mandibular canal (*arrow*). (*C*) Surgical field on the same tooth. (*D*) Postsurgical radiograph.

CBVT has been successfully used to evaluate the position of an instrument fractured in the maxillary sinus between the 2 buccal roots of an upper molar, and to plan orthograde and surgical treatment.[52]

Some authors have even built a CBVT computer-aided design/computer-aided manufacturing guidance system for surgical endodontics.[53]

Orientation Toward a Differential Diagnosis of Lesions of Endodontic Origin

Nonendodontic lesions in the jaws that may need to be differentially diagnosed from AP[54] are lateral periodontal cysts, odontogenic keratocysts, dentigerous cysts, developmental cysts, central giant cell granuloma, traumatic bone cysts, and some forms of ameloblastoma. The differential morphology of radicular cysts, keratocysts, and dentigerous cysts[55] has been described using CT examinations and might help in the diagnosis. Keratocysts and dentigerous cysts can exhibit multilocular or unilocular patterns. Dentigerous cysts are more frequently unilocular, but they are usually in association with the crown of an unerupted tooth.[54] When unilocular, these lesions are more difficult to differentiate from endodontic lesions. On CT, keratocysts and dentigerous cysts tend to develop more into an oval shape and in a direction parallel to the long axis of the mandible. Dentigerous cysts may present with a local expansion of the cortical plate; keratocysts tend to show a discontinuity in the lingual cortex more often than radicular cysts, and are preferably located in the posterior body and ramus of the mandible. Radicular cysts are almost always unilocular, show discontinuity of the lingual cortex of the mandible less often, have a rounder shape, and can be surrounded by a sclerotic bone rim. Giant cell granuloma more often involves the mandible (anterior) and has the radiographic appearance of an irregular radiolucent area that may be unilocular or multilocular, and tends to resorb the roots of the involved teeth. When the lesions are small and unilocular they may simulate AP. They are distinguishable on CT because they are noncorticated (**Fig. 7**).[54]

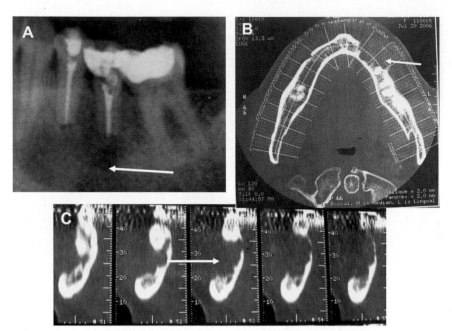

Fig. 7. (A) Panoramic radiograph detail of teeth no. 34 and no. 35 showing a periapical bone lesion (*arrow*). (*B, C*) Dentascan of the same area (*arrows*) showing the extensive involvement of the cortical plates and the scalloping of the bone. The lesion turned out to be a giant cell granuloma.

Nasopalatine canal cysts and static bone cysts (Stafne cyst) are developmental nonodontogenic cysts.[54] The nasopalatine canal cyst on panoramic radiographs is an oval- or heart-shaped radiolucent lesion located between the roots of maxillary central incisors. CT shows an enlargement of the nasopalatine canal on axial or coronal sections. Multiplanar and three-dimensional imaging may be important to show the extent of the lesion.[25,54]

Static bone cyst[54,56] is a depression in the lingual surface of the mandible between its angle and the first molar, below the mandibular canal. The cyst is occasionally found in the anterior mandible. It is caused by aberrant tissue of the submandibular gland, and on CT shows a well-circumscribed radiolucency in the lingual aspect of the mandible with the associated glandular tissue.[56] The traumatic bone cyst is a pseudocyst, probably due to an infrabone hematoma.[54,57] If detected early it contains blood, if later it appears as an empty cavity. On radiographs it is a well-defined radiolucent area, which does not cause interruption of the lamina dura of the teeth involved. On CT (axial scans) it shows expansion with scalloping of the cortical plate and, if present, its fluid content.

The ameloblastoma, more often found in the posterior mandible, appears as a well-defined multilocular or unilocular radiolucent area, which may be associated with resorption or displacement of the roots of the teeth involved. The differential diagnosis of periapical lesions is difficult if the lesion is unilocular. CT shows the expansion of the bone and it becomes important as a differential diagnostic tool in the follow-up of the lesion after an interval of 6 months to 1 year (**Fig. 8**).[54,55] Periapical cemental dysplasia (cemento-osseous dysplastic/reactive lesion) has an initial radiolucent phase, which makes it difficult to be distinguished from periapical lesions. Periapical cemental

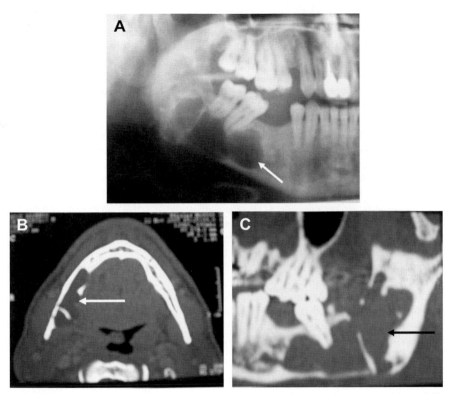

Fig. 8. (*A*) Panoramic radiograph detail of teeth no. 46 and no. 47 showing a wide multiloc-ular bone lesion (*arrow*). (*B, C*) Dentascan of the same area (*arrows*) showing the extensive involvement of the cortical plates and the thinning of the bone. The lesion was an ameloblastoma.

dysplasia is predominantly located in the mandible, and on axial CT scans they show radiopaque masses surrounded by low-density areas with no continuity with the cortical plate and the root of the teeth.[54,58]

When diagnostic doubt refers to the possible presence of a malignancy, then CT is indicated and used in association with contrast media. If the differential diagnosis is between endodontic lesions, then the requirement is to make a distinction between a cyst and a granuloma.[7,8,15] The pioneer application of CT to endodontic lesions came from Trope and colleagues[59] in 1989. These authors selected 8 periapical lesions from human cadavers, which were divided into 4 cysts and 4 granulomas based on the diagnosis made by an oral radiologist. They examined the lesions in the jaws with a CT scan and axial slices, and used a densitometric processor to read the lesions and the surrounding tissues. The CT scan readings were then corre-lated to the histopathology. Of the 8 periapical lesions studied, 7 were granulomas and only 1 was a cyst. It was concluded that cystic cavities could be differentiated from granulomas based on their CT appearance. A cyst on axial CT scans displays an area with a density reading similar to the background, darker than a granuloma or the fibrous tissue of an apical scar. Granuloma has a cloudy appearance with a density similar to that of the surrounding soft tissues. In 1 case, within the same lesion it was possible to distinguish the granulomatous tissue from the cystic cavity inside it.

Controversial reports arise from the application of CBVT to the differential diagnosis of cystic lesions from granulomas. Simon and colleagues[60] examined 17 lesions (1 cm × 1 cm or more) using CVBT to attempt a differential diagnosis between cysts and granulomas based on the measurement of gray values (−4096 gray scale) of the imaged lesion areas. The CBVT diagnosis and the traditional biopsy results coincided only in 13 cases out of 17; 4 cases had a split diagnosis. Frisbie and colleagues[61] used CBVT to make a differential diagnosis between cysts and granulomas in 55 lesions. They based the study on the following parameters: (1) agreement between radiologists as to whether the CBVT image represented a cyst or a granuloma (gray values), (2) agreement between pathologists in deciding if the histopathologic specimen was a cyst or a granuloma, and (3) accuracy of the diagnostic assessment of radiologists using histopathology as the gold standard. The results showed that the pathologists were in high agreement whereas the radiologists were in low agreement and hence, differed in accuracy regarding the diagnosis. The authors concluded that CBVT is not sensitive enough to provide an accurate differential diagnosis among endodontic lesions. Schultze and colleagues[62] reported that CBVT is helpful in the diagnosis of osteomyelitis of the mandible.

Ultrasound real-time echotomography has been used predictably to examine endodontic lesions in the jaws.[63] In an initial study, the differential diagnosis between cystic lesions and granulomas was attempted based on an ultrasound examination complemented by CPD on 11 patients. The patients were diagnosed with periapical lesions and scheduled for endodontic surgery and biopsy. The established criteria to distinguish the 2 lesions were as follows: cyst, annaechoic/transonic, contoured cavity with reinforced walls (pasterior enhancement), fluid content, and no internal vascularization; granuloma, echogenic lesions of different shapes and contours showing vascular supply on CPD.

The provisional echographic diagnosis was compared with the results from the histopathologic examination, which was done after surgical excision of the lesions and semiserial sectioning. The histopathologic reports confirmed the ultrasound diagnosis in all 11 cases. The sensitivity of the technique was particularly enhanced in one case, which showed a mixed echographic appearance, mostly echogenic and vascularized with a well-contoured transonic area in the upper central area. The lesion turned out to be a granuloma containing a small cyst.[64] This study was replicated by a group of researchers who analyzed 15 periapical lesions with echography, conventional and digital radiology, and routine biopsies. Their histology confirmed the ultrasound observations with respect to the underlying lesions, and the authors concluded that ultrasound unequivocally identified the contents and nature of the periapical lesions.[65] A subsequent report on 2 lesions on the same patient, for which the initial diagnosis was done with ultrasound and then validated by the histology confirmed these findings (Figs. 9 and 10).[66] In a more recent paper[67] another 22 radiolucent lesions of the jaws were examined with ultrasound and CPD, and with routine histopathology. The diagnosis of periapical granuloma made with the ultrasound was consistent with the biopsy reports. The lesions that were defined as cysts after the biopsy showed a more varied ultrasound appearance in this report. They were transonic in 5 cases, had a complex and semisolid appearance in 9 specimens (all without internal vascularization), and 1 case appeared as a vascularized solid lesion. Among the lesions histologically classified as cysts there were actually 4 keratocysts, 2 dentigerous cysts, 4 residual cysts, and 7 radicular cysts. These findings might explain why some of the cysts had a mixed fluid and solid content. Furthermore the one cyst that exhibited a solid appearance with internal vascular supply had a very thick capsule and extensive inflammatory content.

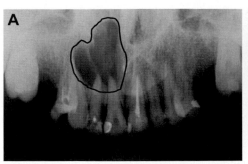
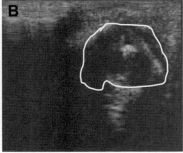

Fig. 9. (A) Panoramic radiograph showing an extensive periapical lesion in the area of teeth no. 11 and no. 12. (B) The ultrasound examination of the area (*circled*) showing a fluid-filled cavity without internal vascularization. The lesion was diagnosed as a cyst.

Ultrasound with CPD can provide accurate information regarding the content of intraosseous lesions of the jaws before surgery, but it does not eliminate the need for a biopsy for histopathologic diagnosis.

Evaluation in Follow-up of the Outcome of Treatment

Periapical radiographs have been used as the gold standard to evaluate healing of endodontic lesions[6,15] and the Periapical Index (PAI) has been used as the scoring system for radiographic assessment of AP.[68] The PAI offers a visual reference scale (scores related to reference radiographs and histologic evaluation of AP) and assigns a health status to the root, based on the changes in the mineral bone content in the periapical area. The score ranges from 1 (absence of pathosis) to 5 (spread of the lesion within the bone) (**Fig. 11**).

In a case report,[48] the authors did the diagnosis and follow-up of an extensive lesion of the maxillary bone using a CT scan and panoramic radiograph. The 18-month follow-up of the panoramic radiograph disclosed a lesion that could be considered healed for about 70% of its extension. The second CT done at the same time showed that the appearance of healing was mostly obtained because the external cortical plate, previously resorbed, had been regenerated. Yet, the size of the lesion was

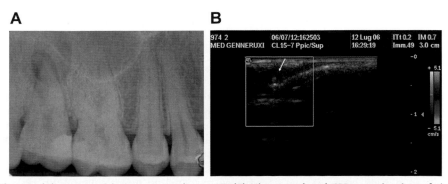

Fig. 10. (A) Periapical lesion on tooth no. 17, (B) Ultrasound and CPD examination of the same lesion (*squared*). The lesion is echogenic and has a rich internal vascularization (*arrow*) and is diagnosed as a granuloma.

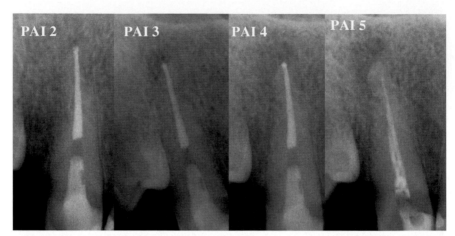

Fig. 11. Representation of the PAI, from the beginning of the pathosis to its spreading in the bone. (The case has been observed in reverse, from the recall to the pretreatment radiograph.)

not reduced to the same extent that could be seen from the radiograph. CT was useful to provide the information on the actual progress of the healing process, which started with the reconstruction of the external cortical plate, and on the necessity to continue to follow-up the case.

Recently, a new PAI system has been developed using criteria established from measurements of periapical lesions as interpreted on CBVT scans, and has been named the CBCT PAI.[44] The index is a scoring system based on the measurement of the lesions in three dimensions (bucco-lingual, mesio-distal, and diagonal) and is determined by the largest extension of that lesion. The scores range from 1 to 6 depending on the largest measure and include the two variables, expansion and destruction of the cortical bone. Radiolucencies measuring more than 8 mm in their largest diameter are given the score 6, whereas 1 is the score for lesions having a larger diameter of 0.5 to 1 mm (**Fig. 12**). The clinical advantages of this system are related to the possibility of assessing the lesions in the 3 planes of space, obtaining more accurate measurements, eliminating false-negative readings, and minimizing the interference of the observers.

With regard to the short-term follow-up of endodontic lesions, in a recent pilot project the authors evaluated the possibility of monitoring the inflammatory changes in diseased bone in response to endodontic treatment. Ultrasound examination associated with CPD was used as a clinical follow-up. In 6 teeth with periapical lesions, the endodontic treatment was completed in 2 appointments using calcium hydroxide as an intermediate medication. Besides periapical radiographs, each case was examined with ultrasound and CPD before treatment (to assess the content of the lesion and its vascularization), 1 week after root canal cleaning and disinfection, and 1 month after the completion of treatment. When the ultrasound/CPD examinations of the same case were compared, a change in the vascularization within the lesions, after the first appointment and after the completion of treatment was observed in all cases. These preliminary data open up new possibilities to follow up endodontic treatment with regard to initial and short-term reactions of lesions at the different stages (and types) of treatment.[69]

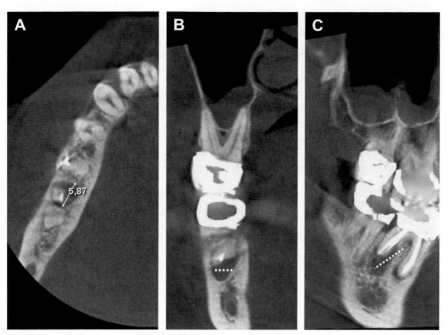

Fig. 12. Representation of CBCT PAI on tooth no. 46, with the measurements of the mesio-distal (*A*), bucco-lingual (*B*), and diagonal diameters (*C*).

SUMMARY

Even if traditional radiology still represents the backbone of everyday endodontic treatment,[6,15] the adjunct of advanced techniques is always indicated when there is a need for more detailed information.[15,25,31] The clinician should be responsible for choosing the most appropriate and convenient examinations for a given investigation. Every time a three-dimensional image is required, either CT or CBVT should be considered. CT is still the best choice for the diagnostic challenges of bone lesions in the jaws. It must be prescribed and used with care to minimize the dose of radiation.[54–59,70] CT can be substituted by CBVT, if available, for most endodontic situations.[25,31] CBVT should not be considered as a substitute for a panoramic radiograph, if this is an adequate examination for a specific case. Not all CBVT investigations and machines dispense the same dose of radiation; some examinations present even more risk than a medical-grade CT.[26–30]

To date, ultrasound imaging is the most sensible technique to address the differential diagnosis of endodontic lesions and to specify their vascular/fluid/solid content in the absence of histopathologic evaluation. It is also valuable for the immediate and short-term clinical follow-up. Ultrasound real-time echotomography is more convenient than computerized tomographs because it entails lower biologic adverse effects.[63–68]

When choosing such advanced imaging techniques the clinician should be aware of and responsible for all the extra information that can be included in these examinations.[25]

Indications on the use of CT for the imaging of AP:

1. Need for predictable information concerning the presence of AP
2. Diagnostic challenges (possible nonodontogenic lesions, different kind of cysts, suspected tumors; need for IV contrast medium)

3. Surgical approach toward very extensive lesions
4. Need for soft tissue examination.

Indications on the use of CBVT for the imaging of AP:

1. Need for predictable information concerning the presence of AP in the jaws
2. Need for additional information useful in the diagnosis and treatment plan of AP (ie, specific roots/teeth involved, additional roots/canals foreign objects, relationship to important anatomic landmarks)
3. Need for specific information on the anatomic coordinates in the surgical approach to endodontic lesions
4. Need for reproducible data for the follow-up of AP (CBCT PAI).

Indications on the use of ultrasound for the imaging of AP:

1. Need for very low risk examination
2. Interest in assessing the content (fluid vs mixed or solid) and vascularization of a lesion
3. Interest in documenting the immediate response to treatment of a lesion (for clinical and scientific purposes).

REFERENCES

1. Torabinejad M, Eby WC, Naidorf IJ. Inflammatory and immunological aspects of the pathogenesis of human periapical lesions. J Endod 1985;11:479–84.
2. Baumgartner JC, Siqueira JR, Sedgley CM, et al. Microbiology of endodontic disease. In: Ingle JI, Bakland LK, Baumgartner JC, editors. Ingle's endodontics. 6th edition. Hamilton (ON): BC Decker Inc; 2008. p. 221–308.
3. Costerton W, Veeh R, Shirtliff M, et al. The application of biofilm science to the study and control of chronic bacterial infections. J Clin Invest 2003;112: 1466–77.
4. Stashenko P, Teles R, D'Souza R. Periradicular inflammatory responses and their modulation. Crit Rev Oral Biol Med 1998;9:498–521.
5. Metzger Z, Abramovitz I. Periapical lesions of endodontic origin. In: Ingle JI, Bakland LK, Baumgartner JC, editors. Ingle's endodontics. 6th edition. Hamilton (ON): BC Decker Inc; 2008. p. 494–519.
6. Huumonen S, Orstavik D. Radiological aspects of apical periodontitis. Endod Top 2002;1:3–25.
7. Simon JH. Incidence of periapical cysts in relation to the root canal. J Endod 1980;6:845–8.
8. Nair PNR. New perspective on radicular cysts: do they heal? Int Endod J 1998;31: 155–60.
9. Nair PNR, Parajola G, Schroeder HE. Types and incidence of human periapical lesions obtained with extracted teeth. Oral Surg Oral Med Oral Pathol Oral Radiol Endod 1996;81:93–102.
10. Nair PNR, Sjogren U, Schumacher E, et al. Radicular cyst affecting a root filled human tooth: a long-term post-treatment follow-up. Int Endod J 1993;26: 225–33.
11. Nair PNR, Sjogren U, Kahnberg KE, et al. Intraradicular bacteria and fungi in root filled, asymptomatic human teeth with therapy-resistant periapical lesions: a long term light and electron microscopy follow-up study. J Endod 1990;16: 580–8.

12. Nair PNR, Sjogren U, Figdor D, et al. Persistent apical radiolucencies of root filed human teeth, failed endodontic treatments and periapical scars. Oral Surg Oral Med Oral Pathol Oral Radiol Endod 1999;87:617–27.
13. Bender IB, Seltzer S. Roentgenographic and direct observation of experimental lesions in bone. J Am Dent Assoc 1961;87:708–16.
14. van der Stelt PF. Experimentally produced bone lesions. Oral Surg Oral Med Oral Pathol Oral Radiol Endod 1985;59:306–12.
15. Cotti E, Campisi G. Advanced radiographic techniques for the detection of lesions in bone. Endod Top 2004;7:52–72.
16. Hounsfield G. Computerized transverse axial scanning (tomography). 1. Description of the system. Br J Radiol 1973;46:1016–22.
17. Abrahams JJ. Dental CT imaging: a look at the jaw. Radiology 2001;219:334–45.
18. Schwarz MS, Rothman SL, Rhodes ML, et al. Computed tomography I. Preoperative assessment of the mandible for endosseous implant surgery. Int J Oral Maxillofac Implants 1987;2:137–41.
19. Schwarz MS, Rothman SL, Rhodes ML, et al. Computed tomography II. Preoperative assessment of the maxilla for endosseous implant surgery. Int J Oral Maxillofac Implants 1987;2:143–8.
20. Pasler FA, Visser H. Computed tomography, radiographic anatomy. In: Pasler FA, Visser H, editors. Pocket atlas of dental radiology. Stuttgart, Germany: Thieme; 2007. p. 98–108.
21. Gahleiter A, Watzek G, Imhof H, et al. Imaging technique, anatomy, and pathological conditions of the jaws. Eur Radiol 2003;13:366–76.
22. Dula K, Mini R, van der Stelt PF, et al. Hypothetical mortality risk associated with spiral computed tomography of the maxilla and mandible. Eur J Oral Sci 1996; 104:503–10.
23. Mozzo P, Procacci C, Tacconi A, et al. A new volumetric CT machine for dental imaging based on the cone-beam technique: preliminary results. Eur Radiol 1998;8:1558–64.
24. Arai Y, Tammisalo E, Iwai K, et al. Development of a compact computed tomographic apparatus for dental use. Dentomaxillofac Radiol 1999;28:245–8.
25. Cotton TP, Geisler TM, Holden DT, et al. Endodontic applications of cone-beam volumetric tomography. J Endod 2007;33:1121–32.
26. Ludlow JB, Davies Ludlow LE, Brooks SL. Dosimetry of two extraoral direct digital imaging devices: NewTom cone beam CT and Orthopos Plus DS panoramic unit. Dentomaxillofac Radiol 2003;32:229–34.
27. Ludlow JB, Davies Ludlow LE, Brooks SL, et al. Dosimetry of 3 CBCT devices for oral and maxillofacial radiology: CB Mercuray, New-Tom 3G and i.CAT. Dentomaxillofac Radiol 2006;35:219–26.
28. Palomo JM, Rao SP, Hans MG. Influence of CBCT exposure condition on radiation dose. Oral Surg Oral Med Oral Pathol Oral Radiol Endod 2008;105:773–82.
29. Hirsh E, Wolf U, Heinicke F, et al. Dosimetry of the cone beam computed tomography Veraviewepocs 3D compared with the 3D Accuitomo in different field of view. Dentomaxillofac Radiol 2008;37:268–73.
30. Loubele M, Jacobs R, Maes F, et al. Image quality vs radiation dose of four cone beam computed tomography scanners. Dentomaxillofac Radiol 2008; 37:309–19.
31. Patel S, Dawood A, Whaites E, et al. New dimensions in endodontic imaging: part 2. Cone beam computed tomography. Int Endod J 2009;42:463–75.
32. Auer LM, Van Velthoven V. Intraoperative ultrasound imaging in neurosurgery. Berlin: Springer Verlag; 1990. p. 1–11.

33. Fleischer A, Emerson DS. Color Doppler sonography in obstetrics and gynae-cology. New York: Churchill Livingstone Inc; 1993. p. 1–32.
34. Martin AO. Can ultrasound cause genetic damage? J Clin Ultrasound 1984;12: 11–20.
35. Barnett SB, Rott HD, Ter Haar GR, et al. The sensitivity of biological tissueto ultra-sound. Ultrasound Med Biol 1997;23:805–12.
36. Barnett SB, Ter Haar GR, Ziskin MC, et al. International recommendations and guidelines for the safe use of diagnostic ultrasound in medicine. Ultrasound Med Biol 2000;20:355–66.
37. Fuhrman R, Bucker A, Diedrich P. Radiological assessment of artificial bone defects in the floor of the maxillary sinus. Dentomaxillofac Radiol 1997;26:112–6.
38. Velvart P, Hecker H, Tillinger G. Detection of the apical lesion and the mandibular canal in conventional radiography and computed radiography. Oral Surg Oral Med Oral Pathol Oral Radiol Endod 2001;2:682–8.
39. Stavropoulos A, Wenzel A. Accuracy of cone beam dental CT, intraoral digital and conventional film radiography for the detection of periapical lesions. En ex vivo study in pig jaws. Clin Oral Investig 2007;11:101–6.
40. Nakata K, Naitoh M, Izumi M, et al. Effectiveness of dental computed radiography in diagnostic imaging of periradicular lesions of each root of a multirooted tooth: a case report. J Endod 2006;32:583–7.
41. Lofthag-Hansen S, Hummonen S, Grondahl K, et al. Limited cone-beam CT and intraoral radiography for the diagnosis of periapical pathology. Oral Surg Oral Med Oral Pathol Oral Radiol Endod 2007;103:114–9.
42. Low KMT, Dula K, Burgin W, et al. Comparison of periapical radiography and limited cone beam tomography in posterior maxillary teeth referred for apical surgery. J Endod 2008;34:557–62.
43. Estrela C, Reis Bueno M, Rodriguez Leles C, et al. Accuracy of cone beam computed tomography and panoramic and periapical radiography for detection of apical periodontitis. J Endod 2008;34:273–9.
44. Estrela C, Reis Bueno M, Correa Azevedo B, et al. A new periapical index based on cone beam computed tomography. J Endod 2008;34:1325–31.
45. Marmary Y, Koter T, Heling I. The effect of periapical rarefying osteitis on cortical and cancellous bone. A study comparing conventional radiographs with computed tomography. Dentomaxillofac Radiol 1999;28:267–71.
46. Eberhardt JH, Torabinejad M, Cjristiansen EL. A computed tomographic study of the distances between the maxillary sinus floor and the apices of maxillary poste-rior teeth. Oral Surg Oral Med Oral Pathol 1992;73:345–6.
47. Rigolone M, Pasqualini D, Bianchi L, et al. Vestibular surgical access to the pala-tine root of the superior first molar: "low dose cone-beam" CT analysis of the pathway and its anatomic variations. J Endod 2003;29:773–5.
48. Cotti E, Vargiu P, Dettori C, et al. Computerized tomography in the management and follow-up of extensive periapical lesion. Endod Dent Traumatol 1999;15: 186–9.
49. Lascala CA, Panella J, Marques MM. Analysis of the accuracy of linear measure-ments obtained by cone beam computed tomography (CBCT-New Tom). Dento-maxillofac Radiol 2004;33:291–4.
50. Ludlow JB, Laster WS, See M, et al. Accuracy of measurements of mandibular anatomy in cone beam computed tomography images. Oral Surg Oral Med Oral Pathol Oral Radiol Endod 2007;103:534–42.
51. Pinsky HM, Dyda S, Pinsky RW, et al. Accuracy of three-dimensional measure-ments using cone-beam CT. Dentomaxillofac Radiol 2006;35:410–6.

52. Tsurumachi T, Honda K. A new cone beam computerized tomography system for use in endodontic surgery. Int Endod J 2007;40:224–32.
53. Pinsky HM, Champleboux G, Sarment DP. Periapical surgery using CAD/CAM guidance: preclinical results. J Endod 2007;33:148–51.
54. DelBalso AM. Lesions of the jaws. Semin Ultrasound CT MR 1995;16:487–512.
55. Yoshiura K, Higuki Y, Araki K, et al. Morphologic analysis of odontogenic cysts with computed tomography. Oral Surg Oral Med Oral Pathol Oral Radiol Endod 1997;83:712–8.
56. Katz J, Chaushu G, Rotstein I. Stafne's bone cavity in the anterior mandible: a possible diagnostic challenge. J Endod 2001;27:304–7.
57. Suei Y, Tanimoto K, Wada T. Simple bone cyst. Evaluation of content with conventional radiography and computed tomography. Oral Surg Oral Med Oral Pathol 1994;77:296–301.
58. Ariji Y, Ariji E, Higuchi Y, et al. Florid cemento-osseous dysplasia. Radiographic study with special emphasis on computed tomography. Oral Surg Oral Med Oral Pathol 1994;78:391–6.
59. Trope M, Pettigrew J, Petras J, et al. Differentiation of periapical granulomas and radicular cysts by digital radiometric analysis. Endod Dent Traumatol 1989;5: 69–72.
60. Simon JHS, Enciso R, Malfaz JM, et al. Differential diagnosis of large periapical lesions using cone beam computed tomography measurements and biopsy. J Endod 2006;32:833–7.
61. Frisbie J, Lee K, Fisch G, et al. Evaluation of pathologists (histopathology) and radiologists (cone beam computed tomography) differentiating periapical cysts from granulomas. J Endod 2009;35:427 (OR 02).
62. Schultze D, Blessman M, Pohlenz P, et al. Diagnostic criteria for the detection of mandibular osteomyelitis using cone–beam computed tomography. Dentomaxillofac Radiol 2006;35:323–5.
63. Cotti E, Campisi G, Garau V, et al. A new technique for the study of periapical bone lesions: ultrasound real time imaging. Int Endod J 2002;35:148–52.
64. Cotti E, Campisi G, Ambu R, et al. Ultrasound real-time imaging in the differential diagnosis of periapical lesions. Int Endod J 2003;36:556–64.
65. Gundappa M, Ng SY, Whaites EJ. Comparison of ultrasound, digital and conventional radiography in differentiating periapical lesions. Dentomaxillofac Radiol 2006;35:326–33.
66. Cotti E, Simbola V, Dettori C, et al. Echographic evaluation of bone lesions of endodontic origin: report of two cases in the same patient. J Endod 2006;32: 901–5.
67. Sumer AP, Danaci M, Ozen Sandikci E, et al. Ultrasonography and Doppler ultrasonography in the evaluation of intraosseous lesions in the jaws. Dentomaxillofac Radiol 2009;38:23–7.
68. Orstavik D, Kerekes K, Eriksen HM. The periapical index: a scoring system for radiographic assessment of apical periodontitis. Endod Dent Traumatol 1986;2: 20–34.
69. Cotti E. Ultrasonic imaging. In: Ingle JI, Bakland LK, Baumgartner JC, editors. Ingle's endodontics. 6th edition. Hamilton (ON): BC Decker Inc; 2008. p. 590–9.
70. Berrington de Gonzales A, Darby S. Risk of cancer from diagnostic X-rays: estimates for the UK and 14 other countries. Lancet 2004;363:345–51.

Local Anesthesia Strategies for the Patient With a "Hot" Tooth

John M. Nusstein, DDS, MS[a],*, Al Reader, DDS, MS[b],
Melissa Drum, DDS, MS[c]

KEYWORDS

• Local anesthesia • Intraosseous injection • Irreversible pulpitis

Achieving profound pulpal anesthesia is a corner stone in endodontic practice and dentistry. Profound pulpal anesthesia during the root canal procedure benefits not only the patient, for obvious reasons, but also the dentist who will be less stressed worrying about patient reactions or sudden movement during therapy. Achieving adequate anesthesia in patients can, at times, be a challenge. But when one adds the condition of a "hot" tooth, the challenges increase. This article describes some strategies that the endodontist can use when treating patients with teeth having moderate-to-severe pain.

To begin, it is necessary to define what a "hot" tooth really is. In endodontic terms, it certainly does not mean a tooth of extreme attractiveness or even a tooth that is undergoing an exothermic reaction in which its temperature is well above normal body temperature. The term "hot" tooth generally refers to a pulp that has been diagnosed with irreversible pulpitis, with spontaneous, moderate-to-severe pain. A classic example of one type of hot tooth is a patient who is sitting in the waiting room, sipping on a large glass of ice water to help control the pain.

Inflammatory changes within the pulp progressively worsen as a carious lesion nears the pulp. Chronic inflammation takes on an acute exacerbation with an influx

Financial disclosure: The authors have no relationship or direct financial interest with any company mentioned in this article. Nor do they have any direct financial interest in the subject matter or materials discussed in this article.
[a] Division of Endodontics, The Ohio State University College of Dentistry, 305 West 12th Avenue, Room 3058, Columbus, OH 43210, USA
[b] Division of Endodontics, The Ohio State University College of Dentistry, 305 West 12th Avenue, Room 3059, Columbus, OH 43210, USA
[c] Department of Endodontics, The Ohio State University College of Dentistry, 305 West 12th Avenue, Room 3059, Columbus, OH 43210, USA
* Corresponding author.
E-mail address: nusstein.1@osu.edu

Dent Clin N Am 54 (2010) 237–247
doi:10.1016/j.cden.2009.12.003
0011-8532/10/$ – see front matter © 2010 Elsevier Inc. All rights reserved.

dental.theclinics.com

of neutrophils and the release of inflammatory mediators (such as prostaglandins and interleukins) and proinflammatory neuropeptides[1] (such as substance P, bradykinin, and calcitonin gene-related peptide). These mediators, in turn, sensitize the peripheral nociceptors within the pulp of the affected tooth, which increases pain production and neuronal excitability.[2] All of this leads to the pain that patients report as they sit in the dental chair.

In dealing with teeth diagnosed with irreversible pulpitis, determining whether adequate local anesthesia has been achieved before treatment is important. Mandibular anesthesia via the inferior alveolar nerve block (IANB) has traditionally been confirmed by asking the patient if their lip feels numb, probing or sticking the gingiva around the mandibular tooth to be treated, or simply starting treatment and waiting for a patient response. However these techniques are not very effective in determining if pulpal anesthesia has been achieved.[3–6] Objective tests can be used to better assess the level of pulpal anesthesia for all teeth. The use of an electric pulp tester (EPT) and/or the application of a cold refrigerant have been shown to accurately determine pulpal anesthesia in teeth with a normal pulp before treatment. If the patient responds negatively to the stimulus (cold or electric current), then pulpal anesthesia has been attained and the patient should not experience pain during treatment. However, in teeth diagnosed with a hot irreversible pulpitis, a failure to respond to the stimulus may not necessarily guarantee pulpal anesthesia.[7–9] The patient may still report pain during treatment. Teeth with necrotic pulp chambers but whose root canals contain vital tissue may not be tested using the above means. In these cases, testing for pulpal anesthesia of the neighboring teeth may give the clinician an indication of the anesthetic status of the tooth to be treated.[9]

When one considers the challenges of local anesthesia in dentistry, mandibular teeth pose the most severe challenge. The IANB must be delivered accurately (indicated by soft tissue and lip numbness) to attain pulpal anesthesia. Missed blocks (lack of lip numbness) occur about 5% of the time and should prompt the provider to re-administer the injection before beginning treatment. When dentists review the literature to determine what injection techniques or anesthetic solutions can offer, they need to be cognizant of the definition of anesthetic success that is used in the research. One way to define anesthetic success for mandibular anesthesia is by the percentage of subjects who achieve 2 consecutive EPT readings of 80 within 15 minutes and sustain these readings for 60 minutes. Clinically, this translates into being able to work on the patient no later than 15 minutes after giving the IANB and having pulpal anesthesia for 1 hour. This duration of anesthesia would be valuable to the endodontist and the restorative dentist. In the available clinical literature it is reported that after administration of a successful IANB (lip numbness achieved) using 2% lidocaine with 1:100,000 epinephrine, success occurs (1) 53% of the time for the mandibular first molar, (2) 61% of the time for the first premolar and (3) 35% of the time for the lateral incisor.[3–6,10–14] Anesthetic failure (the percentage of patients who never achieve 2 consecutive 80 readings with the EPT during 60 minutes of testing) for the mandibular first molar is 17%, 11% for the first premolar, and 32% for the lateral incisor. Patients may also be subject to anesthesia of slow onset. These patients generally do not achieve pulpal anesthesia until after 16 minutes following the IANB, which has been reported to occur in mandibular teeth approximately 19% to 27% of the time, with some patients (8%) having onset after 30 minutes.[3–6,10–14]

When the clinician is confronted with the case of a severe irreversible pulpitis in which the conventional IANB using 2% lidocaine with 1:100,000 epinephrine achieves lip numbness but not pulpal anesthesia (per testing), the question arises as to what strategies can be used to get the patient numb so that the root canal treatment can be done as comfortably as possible.

The first consideration could be to change the local anesthetic agents. Research comparing various local anesthetic agents such as 3% mepivacaine plain (Carbocaine, Polocaine, Scandonest),[4] 4% prilocaine (Citanest Plain),[4] 4% prilocaine with 1:200,000 epinephrine (Citanest Forte),[6] 2% mepivacaine with 1:20,000 levonordefrin (Carbocaine with Neo-Cobefrin),[6] and 4% articaine with 1:100,000 epinephrine (Septocaine)[15] to 2% lidocaine with 1:100,000 epinephrine for the IANB in patients with normal pulps showed that there was no difference in success rates. Therefore, changing local anesthetic agents may not be of benefit. Clinical studies involving patients diagnosed with irreversible pulpitis also failed to show any superiority of 3% mepivacine[16] or 4% articaine with 1:100,000 epinephrine[17] over 2% lidocaine with 1:100,000 epinephrine for the IANB.

The next strategy would be to change the injection technique in attempting to block the inferior alveolar nerve. The Gow-Gates technique[18] has been reported to have a higher success rate than the conventional IANB, but controlled clinical studies have failed to prove its superiority.[19–23] The Vazirani-Akinosi technique (closed mouth) also has not been shown to be superior to the conventional IANB technique.[20,24–26] Therefore, replacing the conventional IANB injection with these techniques will not improve success in attaining pulpal anesthesia in mandibular teeth.

Inaccuracy of the IANB injection has been cited as a contributor to failed mandibular pulpal anesthesia. Hannan and colleagues[10] used medical ultrasound to guide an anesthetic needle to its target for the IANB. They found that although accurate injections could be attained by this method, it did not result in more successful pulpal anesthesia. Therefore, the accuracy of the injection technique (needle placement) was not the primary reason for anesthetic failure with the IANB. Needle deflection as related to the needle bevel direction (toward or away from the mandibular ramus) has also been shown not to affect the anesthetic success rate of the IANB.[27]

Accessory nerves have also been implicated as a potential reason for the failure of the IANB. The incisive nerve block at the mental foramen has been shown to improve anesthetic success of the IANB in first molars and premolars,[28] but the success rate was not as good as other supplemental anesthetic techniques. The mylohyoid nerve is the accessory nerve most often implicated as the cause for mandibular anesthesia failure.[29,30] However, Clark and colleagues,[31] when combining the IANB with a mylohyoid injection after locating the mylohyoid nerve with a peripheral nerve stimulator, found no significant improvement in mandibular anesthesia when the mylohyoid injection was added.

Increasing the volume of the local anesthetic delivered during the IANB has also been found not to increase the incidence of pulpal anesthesia.[3,14,31–33] Increasing the concentration of epinephrine (1:50,000), with the hopes of keeping the anesthetic agent at the injection site longer, also showed no advantage in the IANB.[11,34]

So why then is it so difficult to achieve adequate pulpal anesthesia in mandibular teeth, even if the patient is asymptomatic? The central core theory may be the best explanation.[35,36] This theory states that the outer nerves of the inferior alveolar nerve bundle supply the molar teeth, whereas the nerves for the anterior teeth lie deeper. Anesthetic solutions that are currently used may not be able to diffuse into the nerve trunk to reach all the nerves and provide an adequate block, which explains the difficulty in achieving successful anesthesia for mandibular anterior teeth.[2–6,10–14,19]

Patients in pain as a result of a tooth diagnosed with irreversible pulpitis have additional difficulties attaining pulpal anesthesia. One theory to explain this is that the inflamed tissue has a lowered pH, which reduces the amount of the base form of the anesthetic needed to penetrate the nerve sheath and membrane. Therefore, there is less ionized form of the anesthetic within the nerve to produce anesthesia. This theory may explain only the local effects of inflammation on the nerve and not why an IANB injection is less successful when given at a distance from the area of inflammation (the hot tooth). Another theory is that the nerves arising from the inflamed tissue have altered resting potentials and reduced thresholds of excitability.[37,38] It was shown that anesthetic agents were not able to prevent the transmission of nerve impulses because of the lowered excitability thresholds[37,39] of inflamed nerves. Other theories have looked at the presence of anesthetic-resistant sodium channels[40] and the upregulation of sodium channels in pulps diagnosed with irreversible pulpitis.[41]

SUPPLEMENTAL INJECTIONS

Failure of the traditional IANB in asymptomatic and symptomatic patients requires that a clinician have fall-back strategies to attain good pulpal anesthesia, especially when a patient complains of pain too severe for the clinician to proceed with treatment, as is often the case of patients with hot teeth. There are several supplemental injection techniques available to help the dentist/endodontist, which are reviewed in this article. It should be reiterated that these supplemental techniques are used best after attaining a clinically successful IANB (lip numbness).

Intraligamentary (Periodontal Ligament) Injection

Bangerter and colleagues[42] reported that the periodontal ligament (PDL) supplemental injection is still one of the most widely taught and used supplemental techniques. The success of supplemental PDL injections in helping achieve anesthesia for endodontic procedures has been reported to be 50% to 96%.[16,43,44] Often reinjection is required because of failure of the initial PDL injection. Walton and Abbott[43] reported an initial success rate of 71%, and when reinjection was used, the overall success rate was 92%. Smith and colleagues[44] also reported an increase in success when a second PDL injection was required. In patients with irreversible pulpitis, Cohen and colleagues[16] reported that the supplemental PDL injections were successful 74% of the time, whereas reinjection boosted success to 96%. The key to giving a successful PDL injection remains the attainment of back-pressure during the injection.[43,45] Failure to get back-pressure will most likely lead to failure.[43,46]

PDL injections are usually given using either a standard dental anesthetic syringe or a high-pressure syringe. The development of computer-controlled anesthetic delivery systems (the Wand or the Single Tooth Anesthesia [Milestone Scientific, Livingston, NJ, USA] devices) have been found to be able to deliver a PDL injection. Berlin and colleagues,[47] using the Wand, found that with a primary PDL injection, successful anesthesia (2 consecutive 80/80 readings) was attained in mandibular first molars 86% of the time with 4% articaine with 1:100,000 epinephrine and 74% of the time with 2% lidocaine with 1:100,000 epinephrine. No significant difference was found between the 2 solutions. The Wand system was able to deliver 1.4 mL of the anesthetic over the course of the injection. When this system was used, the duration of anesthesia for the first molar averaged from 31 to 34 minutes, which was longer than the 10 minutes reported by White and colleagues[48] when they used a pressure syringe and delivered only 0.4 mL of 2% lidocaine with 1:100,000 epinephrine. No research on the Single Tooth Anesthesia device is currently available for review.

In patients diagnosed with irreversible pulpitis and experiencing moderate-to-severe pain, when a supplemental PDL injection was delivered using the Wand, the rate of success of the injection was 56%.[49] Success in this study was defined as no pain or mild pain on access and instrumentation of the canals of the affected tooth. The PDL injections used 2% lidocaine with 1:100,000 epinephrine and were limited to mandibular posterior teeth after successful IANB injections (lip numbness only).

Intraosseous Injection

The use of the intraosseous (IO) injection allows the practitioner to deliver local anesthetic solutions directly into the cancellous bone surrounding the affected tooth. There are several IO systems available in the market, including the Stabident system (Fairfax Dental Inc, Wimbledon, UK), X-Tip system (Dentsply, York, PA, USA), and IntraFlow handpiece (Pro-Dex Inc, Santa Ana, CA, USA). The Stabident system consists of a 27-gauge beveled wire that is driven by a slow-speed handpiece, which perforates the cortical bone. Anesthetic solution is then delivered into the cancellous bone with a 27-gauge ultrashort needle through the perforation using a standard anesthetic syringe. The X-Tip system consists of a 2-part perforator/guide sleeve component, which is also driven by a slow-speed handpiece. The perforator leads the guide sleeve through the cortical bone and then is separated from it and removed. This leaves the guide sleeve in place and allows for a 27-gauge needle to be inserted for injecting the anesthetic solution. The guide sleeve is then removed with a hemostat at the end of the appointment. The IntraFlow handpiece holds and drives a perforating needle and an anesthetic cartridge, which is engaged via an internal clutch to deliver the local anesthetic through the perforation.

One of the benefits of the IO injection is the reported immediate onset of anesthesia.[50–58] The injection is recommended to be given distal to the tooth to be anesthetized.[50–58] The exception to this rule would be the maxillary and mandibular second molars, for which a mesial site injection would be needed. The perforation site for the IO injection should be equidistant between the teeth and in the attached gingiva to allow for the perforation to be made through a minimal thickness of tissue and cortical bone and to prevent damage to the roots of the teeth. Perforation in the attached tissue also allows for easier location of the perforation site with the Stabident system. The X-Tip could be used in a more apical area below the mucogingival junction if needed because the guide sleeve remains in place and therefore, there is no difficulty in locating the perforation hole. This may also be attempted with the IntraFlow system. The apical location of the injection would be advisable if the patient has no attached tissue around the affected tooth, if there is a lack of interproximal space between adjacent roots, or if the Stabident IO injection did not achieve adequate anesthesia.

Research on the supplemental IO injection for patients diagnosed with irreversible pulpitis has shown good results. Nusstein and colleagues[8] found that a supplemental mandibular IO injection using 1.8 mL of 2% lidocaine with 1:100,000 epinephrine had a 91% success rate in attaining complete pulpal anesthesia when used after the IANB injection failed. Parente and colleagues[59] reported a success rate of 79% when they used 0.45 to 0.9 mL of 2% lidocaine with 1:100,000 epinephrine. The addition of a second IO injection increased their reported success to 91%. Reisman and colleagues[60] used 1.8 mL of 3% mepivacaine as a supplemental injection in mandibular, posterior teeth diagnosed with irreversible pulpitis. They reported 80% success with an initial IO injection and 98% success when a second IO injection of mepivacaine was delivered. Bigby and colleagues[61] studied 4% articaine with 1:100,000 epinephrine as an IO supplemental injection in posterior mandibular teeth diagnosed with irreversible pulpitis and reported an 86% success rate when the IANB injection failed. The Stabident system was used in all these 4 studies.

Using the X-Tip system for the supplemental IO injection in patients diagnosed with irreversible pulpitis, Nusstein and colleagues[50] reported an 82% success rate when using 1.8 mL of 2% lidocaine with 1:100,000 epinephrine in mandibular posterior teeth. In this study, the injection site was 3 to 7 mm apical to the mucogingival junction. The failures of the injection were attributed to backflow of the anesthetic out of the guide sleeve during the injection. This backflow usually indicates an incomplete perforation or blockage of the guide sleeve. Remmers and colleagues[62] used the IntraFlow system as a primary IO injection in 15 patients diagnosed with irreversible pulpitis and reported an 87% success rate. Their definition of success was 2 consecutive 80/80 readings with the EPT. They reported that failures were because of clogging of the perforating needle and subsequent leakage of the anesthetic around the transducer assembly. However, the study sampled a very small number of patients, and further research is needed on the Intraflow system.

The duration of anesthesia for a supplemental IO injection in patients with irreversible pulpitis has been reported to last the entire debridement appointment of approximately 45 minutes.[8,49,60] The duration will be shorter with the 3% mepivacaine solution.[59]

One of the concerns when using the IO injection is the reported transient increase in heart rate with both the Stabident and X-Tip systems when injecting epinephrine- and levonordefrin-containing anesthetic solutions.[8,50–57,61,63] Replogle and colleagues[63] reported that 67% of subjects had an increase in heart rate as measured on an electrocardiograph when 1.8 mL of 2% lidocaine with 1:100,000 epinephrine was used. The increase in heart rate ranged from 12 to 32 beats per minute.[51,53,61,63,64] The use of 3% mepivacaine has been reported not to cause any significant increase in the heart rate[63,65] and may be an excellent alternative when a patient's medical history or drug therapies contraindicate the use of epinephrine or levonordefrin.

Mandibular Buccal Infiltration Injection with Articaine

Recent research has looked at the use of a mandibular buccal infiltration injection of 4% articaine with 1:100,000 epinephrine as a supplemental injection to increase the success of the IANB injection. In asymptomatic patients, the use of the articaine solution was found to be superior to the lidocaine solution (88% vs 71%, respectively, when success was defined as achieving 2 consecutive readings of 80 with the EPT and maintaining anesthesia for 60 minutes).[66] Kanaa and colleagues[67] reported a success rate of 91% (2 consecutive readings of 80 during the test period) with 4% articaine with 1:100,000 epinephrine. However, when the buccal infiltration injection was used as a supplement to the IANB in patients diagnosed with irreversible pulpitis, success was reported as only 58%.[68] This result was much less than that attained with the IO and PDL injections.

Intrapulpal Injection

In approximately 5% to 10% of mandibular teeth diagnosed with irreversible pulpitis, supplemental injections (PDL and IO) do not produce adequate anesthesia, even when repeated, to enter the pulp chamber painlessly. This is a prime indication that an intrapulpal injection may be necessary.

The intrapulpal injection works well when it is given under back-pressure.[69,70] Onset of anesthesia is immediate. Various techniques have been advocated in giving the injection; however, the key factor is giving the injection under strong back-pressure. Simply placing local anesthetic solution in the pulp chamber will not achieve adequate pulpal anesthesia.

A disadvantage of the intrapulpal injection is its short duration of action (approximately 15–20 minutes). Once anesthesia is achieved, the practitioner must work quickly to remove all the tissue from the pulp chamber and the canals. The intrapulpal injection also requires that the pulp tissue be exposed to permit the injection to be given. Achieving a pulpal exposure could be very painful to the patient because the pain of treatment may begin when the dentin is exposed.[8,50,60,61,70] The injection can be very painful for the patient. The patient should be warned to expect moderate to severe pain during the initial phase of the injection.

Preemptive Strategies to Improve Success of the IANB Injection

Recent clinical studies have looked at the use of oral medications before treatment of a patient with a tooth diagnosed with irreversible pulpitis in hopes of improving the success rate of the IANB injection. Ianiro and colleagues[71] used pretreatment oral doses of acetaminophen or a combination of acetaminophen and ibuprofen versus placebo in patients undergoing endodontic therapy. They reported a trend toward higher success rates (defined as no pain upon entering the pulp chamber) of 71% to 76%, respectively, as compared with placebo (46%). These differences, however, were not found to be significant. Galatin and colleagues[72] used an IO injection of 40 mg of methylprednisolone (Depo-Medrol) and found that it significantly reduced pain and use of medication in untreated patients diagnosed with irreversible pulpitis when compared with patients who received a placebo injection. Unfortunately, follow-up studies by Agarwala and colleagues[73] and Stein and colleagues[74] using similar doses of methylprednisolone failed to improve the success of the IANB injection.

Anxiety is believed to play a role in lowering pain thresholds, and the use of a sedative agent to help increase the success of the IANB injection in patients diagnosed with irreversible pulpitis was studied by Lindemann and colleagues[75] This group used sublingual triazolam and found that a dose of 0.25 mg given 30 minutes before treatment failed to improve the success rate of the IANB as compared with placebo. They concluded that, with conscious sedation, profound pulpal anesthesia was still required to eliminate pain during endodontic treatment of a hot tooth.

SUMMARY

The dentist who treats patients diagnosed with a mandibular hot tooth (irreversible pulpitis) will often find achieving adequate pulpal anesthesia to be a challenge. It behooves each provider to develop a plan to deal with the eventual failures found with the IANB injection. This plan needs to include the use of supplemental anesthesia techniques. Whether the clinician's training or preference is the PDL or IO injection, these supplemental techniques have been shown to be quite effective in achieving pulpal anesthesia for teeth with irreversible pulpitis. Being able to fall back on both sets of techniques provides the dentist the confidence to provide relatively pain-free treatment for the patient having a hot tooth.

REFERENCES

1. Byers MR, Närhi MV. Dental injury models: experimental tools for understanding neuroinflammatory interactions and polymodal nociceptor functions. Crit Rev Oral Biol Med 1999;10(1):4–39.
2. Dray A. Inflammatory mediators of pain. Br J Anaesth 1995;75(2):125–31.
3. Vreeland DL, Reader A, Beck M, et al. An evaluation of volumes and concentrations of lidocaine in human inferior alveolar nerve block. J Endod 1989;15(1): 6–12.

4. McLean C, Reader A, Beck M, et al. An evaluation of 4% prilocaine and 3% mepivacaine compared with 2% lidocaine (1:100,000 epinephrine) for inferior alveolar nerve block. J Endod 1993;19(3):146–50.
5. Chaney MA, Kerby R, Reader A, et al. An evaluation of lidocaine hydrocarbonate compared with lidocaine hydrochloride for inferior alveolar nerve block. Anesth Prog 1991;38(6):212–6.
6. Hinkley SA, Reader A, Beck M, et al. An evaluation of 4% prilocaine with 1:200,000 epinephrine and 2% mepivacaine with 1:20,000 levonordefrin compared with 2% lidocaine with:100,000 epinephrine for inferior alveolar nerve block. Anesth Prog 1991;38(3):84–9.
7. Dreven LJ, Reader A, Beck M, et al. An evaluation of an electric pulp tester as a measure of analgesia in human vital teeth. J Endod 1987;13(5):233–8.
8. Nusstein J, Reader A, Nist R, et al. Anesthetic efficacy of the supplemental intra-osseous injection of 2% lidocaine with 1:100,000 epinephrine in irreversible pulpitis. J Endod 1998;24(7):487–91.
9. Hsiao-Wu GW, Susarla SM, White RR. Use of the cold test as a measure of pulpal anesthesia during endodontic therapy: a randomized, blinded, placebo-controlled clinical trial. J Endod 2007;33(4):406–10.
10. Hannan L, Reader A, Nist R, et al. The use of ultrasound for guiding needle place-ment for inferior alveolar nerve blocks. Oral Surg Oral Med Oral Pathol Oral Radiol Endod 1999;87(6):658–65.
11. Wali M, Reader A, Beck M, et al. Anesthetic efficacy of lidocaine and epinephrine in human alveolar nerve blocks. J Endod 1988;14(4):193.
12. Simon F, Reader A, Meyer W, et al. Evaluation of a peripheral nerve stimulator in human mandibular anesthesia. J Dent Res 1990;69(3):304.
13. Fernandez C, Reader A, Beck M, et al. A prospective, randomized, double-blind comparison of bupivacaine and lidocaine for inferior alveolar nerve blocks. J Endod 2005;31(7):499–503.
14. Nusstein J, Reader A, Beck M. Anesthetic efficacy of different volumes of lidocaine with epinephrine for inferior alveolar nerve blocks. Gen Dent 2002;50(4):372–5.
15. Mikesell P, Nusstein J, Reader A, et al. A comparison of articaine and lidocaine for inferior alveolar nerve blocks. J Endod 2005;31(4):265–70.
16. Cohen H, Cha B, Spångberg L. Endodontic anesthesia in mandibular molars: a clinical study. J Endod 1993;19(7):370–3.
17. Claffey E, Reader A, Nusstein J, et al. Anesthetic efficacy of articaine for inferior alveolar nerve blocks in patients with irreversible pulpitis. J Endod 2004;30(8):568–71.
18. Gow-Gates GA. Mandibular conduction anesthesia: a new technique using extraoral landmarks. Oral Surg Oral Med Oral Pathol 1973;36(3):321–8.
19. Agren E, Danielsson K. Conduction block analgesia in the mandible. A compar-ative investigation of the techniques of Fischer and Gow-Gates. Swed Dent J 1981;5(3):81–9.
20. Todorović L, Stajcić Z, Petrović V. Mandibular versus inferior dental anaesthesia: clinical assessment of 3 different techniques. Int J Oral Maxillofac Surg 1986;15(6):733–8.
21. Goldberg S, Reader A, Drum M, et al. Comparison of the anesthetic efficacy of the conventional inferior alveolar, Gow-Gates, and Vazirani-Akinosi techniques. J Endod 2008;34(11):1306–11.
22. Montagnese T, Reader A, Melfi R. A comparative study of the Gow-Gates tech-nique and a standard technique for mandibular anesthesia. J Endod 1984;10(4):158–63.

23. Hung P, Chang H, Yang P, et al. Comparison of the Gow-Gates mandibular block and inferior alveolar nerve block using a standardized protocol. J Formos Med Assoc 2006;105(2):139–46.
24. Sisk A. Evaluation of the Akinosi mandibular block technique in oral surgery. J Oral Maxillofac Surg 1986;44(2):113–5.
25. Yücel E, Hutchison I. A comparative evaluation of the conventional and closed-mouth technique for inferior alveolar nerve block. Aust Dent J 1995;40(1):15–6.
26. Martínez González J, Benito Peña B, Fernández Cáliz F, et al. A comparative study of direct mandibular nerve block and the Akinosi technique. Med Oral 2003;8(2):143–9.
27. Steinkruger G, Nusstein J, Reader A, et al. The significance of needle bevel orientation in achieving a successful inferior alveolar nerve block. J Am Dent Assoc 2006;137(12):1685–91.
28. Nist R, Reader A, Beck M, et al. An evaluation of the incisive nerve block and combination inferior alveolar and incisive nerve blocks in mandibular anesthesia. J Endod 1992;18(9):455–9.
29. Frommer J, Mele F, Monroe C. The possible role of the mylohyoid nerve in mandibular posterior tooth sensation. J Am Dent Assoc 1972;85(1):113–7.
30. Wilson S, Johns P, Fuller P. The inferior alveolar and mylohyoid nerves: an anatomic study and relationship to local anesthesia of the anterior mandibular teeth. J Am Dent Assoc 1984;108(3):350–2.
31. Clark S, Reader A, Beck M, et al. Anesthetic efficacy of the mylohyoid nerve block and combination inferior alveolar nerve block/mylohyoid nerve block. Oral Surg Oral Med Oral Pathol Oral Radiol Endod 1999;87(5):557–63.
32. Yared G, Dagher F. Evaluation of lidocaine in human inferior alveolar nerve block. J Endod 1997;23(9):575–8.
33. Yonchak T, Reader A, Beck M, et al. Anesthetic efficacy of unilateral and bilateral inferior alveolar nerve blocks to determine cross innervation in anterior teeth. Oral Surg Oral Med Oral Pathol Oral Radiol Endod 2001;92(2):132–5.
34. Dagher F, Yared G, Machtou P. An evaluation of 2% lidocaine with different concentrations of epinephrine for inferior alveolar nerve block. J Endod 1997;23(3):178–80.
35. de Jong R. Neural blockade by local anesthetics. JAMA 1977;238(13):1383–5.
36. Strichartz GR. Molecular mechanisms of nerve block by local anesthesics. Anesth 1976;45(4):421–44.
37. Wallace J, Michanowicz A, Mundell R, et al. A pilot study of the clinical problem of regionally anesthetizing the pulp of an acutely inflamed mandibular molar. Oral Surg Oral Med Oral Pathol 1985;59(5):517–21.
38. Byers M, Taylor P, Khayat B, et al. Effects of injury and inflammation on pulpal and periapical nerves. J Endod 1990;16(2):78–84.
39. Modaresi J, Dianat O, Soluti A. Effect of pulp inflammation on nerve impulse quality with or without anesthesia. J Endod 2008;34(4):438–41.
40. Roy M, Narahashi T. Differential properties of tetrodotoxin-sensitive and tetrodotoxin-resistant sodium channels in rat dorsal root ganglion neurons. J Neurosci 1992;12(6):2104–11.
41. Sorensen H, Skidmore L, Rzasa D, et al. Comparison of pulpal sodium channel density in normal teeth to diseased teeth with severe spontaneous pain. J Endod 2004;30(4):287.
42. Bangerter C, Mines P, Sweet M. The use of intraosseous anesthesia among endodontists: results of a questionnaire. J Endod 2009;35(1):15–8.
43. Walton R, Abbott B. Periodontal ligament injection: a clinical evaluation. J Am Dent Assoc 1981;103(4):571–5.

44. Smith G, Walton R, Abbott B. Clinical evaluation of periodontal ligament anesthesia using a pressure syringe. J Am Dent Assoc 1983;107(6):953–6.
45. Smith G, Walton R. Periodontal ligament injection: distribution of injected solutions. Oral Surg Oral Med Oral Pathol 1983;55(3):232–8.
46. Malamed S. Supplemental injection techniques. In: Handbook of local anesthesia. 5th edition. St. Louis (MO): Elsivier Mosby; 2004. p. 255–68.
47. Berlin J, Nusstein J, Reader A, et al. Efficacy of articaine and lidocaine in a primary intraligamentary injection administered with a computer-controlled local anesthetic delivery system. Oral Surg Oral Med Oral Pathol Oral Radiol Endod 2005;99(3):361–6.
48. White J, Reader A, Beck M, et al. The periodontal ligament injection: a comparison of the efficacy in human maxillary and mandibular teeth. J Endod 1988;14(10):508–14.
49. Nusstein J, Claffey E, Reader A, et al. Anesthetic effectiveness of the supplemental intraligamentary injection, administered with a computer-controlled local anesthetic delivery system, in patients with irreversible pulpitis. J Endod 2005; 31(5):354–8.
50. Nusstein J, Kennedy S, Reader A, et al. Anesthetic efficacy of the supplemental X-tip intraosseous injection in patients with irreversible pulpitis. J Endod 2003; 29(11):724–8.
51. Guglielmo A, Reader A, Nist R, et al. Anesthetic efficacy and heart rate effects of the supplemental intraosseous injection of 2% mepivacaine with 1:20,000 levonordefrin. Oral Surg Oral Med Oral Pathol Oral Radiol Endod 1999;87(3):284–93.
52. Dunbar D, Reader A, Nist R, et al. Anesthetic efficacy of the intraosseous injection after an inferior alveolar nerve block. J Endod 1996;22(9):481–6.
53. Stabile P, Reader A, Gallatin E, et al. Anesthetic efficacy and heart rate effects of the intraosseous injection of 1.5% etidocaine (1:200,000 epinephrine) after an inferior alveolar nerve block. Oral Surg Oral Med Oral Pathol Oral Radiol Endod 2000;89(4):407–11.
54. Coggins R, Reader A, Nist R, et al. Anesthetic efficacy of the intraosseous injection in maxillary and mandibular teeth. Oral Surg Oral Med Oral Pathol Oral Radiol Endod 1996;81(6):634–41.
55. Gallatin J, Reader A, Nusstein J, et al. A comparison of two intraosseous anesthetic techniques in mandibular posterior teeth. J Am Dent Assoc 2003;134(11):1476–84.
56. Reitz J, Reader A, Nist R, et al. Anesthetic efficacy of the intraosseous injection of 0.9 mL of 2% lidocaine (1:100,000 epinephrine) to augment an inferior alveolar nerve block. Oral Surg Oral Med Oral Pathol Oral Radiol Endod 1998;86(5): 516–23.
57. Reitz J, Reader A, Nist R, et al. Anesthetic efficacy of a repeated intraosseous injection given 30 min following an inferior alveolar nerve block/intraosseous injection. Anesth Prog 1998;45(4):143–9.
58. Replogle K, Reader A, Nist R, et al. Anesthetic efficacy of the intraosseous injection of 2% lidocaine (1:100,000 epinephrine) and 3% mepivacaine in mandibular first molars. Oral Surg Oral Med Oral Pathol Oral Radiol Endod 1997;83(1):30–7.
59. Parente S, Anderson R, Herman W, et al. Anesthetic efficacy of the supplemental intraosseous injection for teeth with irreversible pulpitis. J Endod 1998;24(12):826–8.
60. Reisman D, Reader A, Nist R, et al. Anesthetic efficacy of the supplemental intraosseous injection of 3% mepivacaine in irreversible pulpitis. Oral Surg Oral Med Oral Pathol Oral Radiol Endod 1997;84(6):676–82.
61. Bigby J, Reader A, Nusstein J, et al. Anesthetic efficacy of lidocaine/meperidine for inferior alveolar nerve blocks in patients with irreversible pulpitis. J Endod 2007;33(1):7–10.

62. Remmers T, Glickman G, Spears R, et al. The efficacy of IntraFlow intraosseous injection as a primary anesthesia technique. J Endod 2008;34(3):280–3.
63. Replogle K, Reader A, Nist R, et al. Cardiovascular effects of intraosseous injections of 2 percent lidocaine with 1:100,000 epinephrine and 3 percent mepivacaine. J Am Dent Assoc 1999;130(5):649–57.
64. Chamberlain T, Davis R, Murchison D, et al. Systemic effects of an intraosseous injection of 2% lidocaine with 1:100,000 epinephrine. Gen Dent 2000;48(3): 299–302.
65. Gallatin E, Stabile P, Reader A, et al. Anesthetic efficacy and heart rate effects of the intraosseous injection of 3% mepivacaine after an inferior alveolar nerve block. Oral Surg Oral Med Oral Pathol Oral Radiol Endod 2000;89(1):83–7.
66. Haase A, Reader A, Nusstein J, et al. Comparing anesthetic efficacy of articaine versus lidocaine as a supplemental buccal infiltration of the mandibular first molar after an inferior alveolar nerve block. J Am Dent Assoc 2008;139(9):1228–35.
67. Kanaa M, Whitworth J, Corbett I, et al. Articaine buccal infiltration enhances the effectiveness of lidocaine inferior alveolar nerve block. Int Endod J 2009;42(3): 238–46.
68. Matthews R, Drum M, Reader A, et al. Articaine for supplemental buccal mandibular infiltration anesthesia in patients with irreversible pulpitis when the inferior alveolar nerve block fails. J Endod 2009;35(3):343–6.
69. Birchfield J, Rosenberg P. Role of the anesthetic solution in intrapulpal anesthesia. J Endod 1975;1(1):26–7.
70. VanGheluwe J, Walton R. Intrapulpal injection: factors related to effectiveness. Oral Surg Oral Med Oral Pathol Oral Radiol Endod 1997;83(1):38–40.
71. Ianiro S, Jeansonne B, McNeal S, et al. The effect of preoperative acetaminophen or a combination of acetaminophen and Ibuprofen on the success of inferior alveolar nerve block for teeth with irreversible pulpitis. J Endod 2007;33(1):11–4.
72. Gallatin E, Reader A, Nist R, et al. Pain reduction in untreated irreversible pulpitis using an intraosseous injection of Depo-Medrol. J Endod 2000;26(11):633–8.
73. Agarwala V, Reader A, Nusstein J, et al. Anesthetic effect of a preemptive intraosseous injection of Depo-Medrol in untreated irreversible pulpitis. J Endod 2006; 32(3):238.
74. Stein K, Reader A, Agarwala V, et al. Anesthetic effectiveness of a preemptive injection of Depo-Medrol in untreated irreversible pulpitis. J Endod 2007;33(3): 332.
75. Lindemann M, Reader A, Nusstein J, et al. Effect of sublingual triazolam on the success of inferior alveolar nerve block in patients with irreversible pulpitis. J Endod 2008;34(10):1167–70.

Modern Molar Endodontic Access and Directed Dentin Conservation

David Clark, DDS[a],*, John Khademi, DDS, MS[b]

KEYWORDS

• Molar • Endodontic • Access • Dentin

During patient treatment, the clinician needs to consider many factors that will affect the ultimate outcome. In simple terms, these factors can be grouped into 3 categories: the operator needs, the restoration needs, and the tooth needs. The operator needs are the conditions the clinician needs to treat the tooth. The restoration needs are the prep dimensions and tooth conditions for optimal strength and longevity. The tooth needs are the biologic and structural limitations for a treated tooth to remain predictably functional. This article discusses molar access and failures of endodontically treated teeth that occur not because of chronic or acute apical lesions but because of structural compromises to the teeth that ultimately renders them useless. What both authors have discovered in their respective practices through careful observations of failing cases and modes of failure, and observation of the truly long-term (decades) successful cases, is that the current models of endodontic treatment do not lead to long-term success. The authors want to coronally shift the focus to the cervical area of the tooth and create awareness for an endorestorative interface. This article introduces a set of criteria that will guide the clinician in treatment decisions to maintain optimal functionality of the tooth and help in deciding whether the treatment prognosis is poor and alternatives should be considered. This article is not an update on traditional endodontic access, as the authors believe the traditional approach to endodontic access is fundamentally flawed. Traditional endodontic access has been endodontic centric, primarily focused on operator needs, and has been decoupled from the restorative needs and tooth needs. Central to our philosophy is that balance needs to be restored to these 3 needs, which are almost always in conflict when performing complete cusp-tip to root-tip treatment.

Disclosure: Drs Clark and Khademi will receive a royalty from the sales of CK Endodontic Access burs. http://www.sswhiteburs.com.
[a] 3402 South 38th Street, Tacoma, WA 98409, USA
[b] 2277 West 2nd Avenue, Durango, CO 81301-4658, USA
* Corresponding author.
E-mail address: drclark@microscopedentistry.com

Dent Clin N Am 54 (2010) 249–273
doi:10.1016/j.cden.2010.01.001
0011-8532/10/$ – see front matter © 2010 Elsevier Inc. All rights reserved.

dental.theclinics.com

SETTING THE STAGE FOR CONTEMPORARY MOLAR ENDODONTIC ACCESS

Modern clinicians must factor the unique and dramatically higher biting force of the molar tooth when designing the endodontic portion of the endo-endorestorative-prosthodontic (EERP) continuum. The occlusal forces created by the attachment position of the elevator muscles to the mandible generate occlusal forces that vary dramatically throughout the dentition, with light biting force in the front of the mouth to increasingly heavier forces at the back of the mouth. In physics, the mandible with its hinged access (the temporomandibular joint) is classified as a moment arm. The closer to the hinge, the higher the moment, or force, applied. The ability of the incisor to splay forward when loaded occlusally also comes into play when evaluating tooth stresses during occlusal loading. However, the molar absorbs a more vertical force and, therefore, a significantly higher net compressive force. When these 2 factors are combined (moment arm and splay), the overall compressive forces on the molar create a situation that requires a different set of rules for the calculation of ferrule, post and core design, resistance to fracturing, and (of utmost importance) endodontic access and removal of radicular dentin during endodontic shaping.

There are also different forces. The incisor must withstand milder, but more oblique, shearing forces. Most of the in vitro and in vivo research of post and core design has been conducted on maxillary incisor teeth, and attempting to extrapolate these findings to the molar tooth is not feasible. Placing a post in a round, husky maxillary anterior root and subjecting it to mild shearing force has little relevance to placing a post in a delicate, ovoid root in a mandibular molar and subjecting it to heavy compressive force.

Box 1 presents a compelling argument for change, or, perhaps, a return to the pre-Schilder era of directed dentin conservation. Many people were hopeful that the promise of point number 1, the endodontic monoblock of bonded endodontic obturants, posts, and cores, could revitalize a hollowed-out tooth. This has not reached fruition. Most restorative dentists are unaware of point number 2. Most have always assumed that coronal composite restorations, especially those that are bonded to enamel, strengthen the crown of the tooth and prevent coronal fracturing. This common notion has created a false hope, as no such intracoronal splinting benefit exists. Point number 4 eliminates posts as a reconstructive asset in molars. Point 5 presents the troubling fact that altering the thickness of radicular dentin, especially in the ovoid and fluted root, predisposes the root to fracture. Yet the dentin in the endodontically treated tooth has virtually the same strength and moisture content as a tooth with intact pulp. Root fractures in endodontically treated teeth should be considered as iatrogenically generated, not because of any fault of the tooth. The authors have exhausted the means to reinforce the endodontically treated molar stump, and now realize that dentin is the key.

Box 1
Current research and restorative trends

(1) The failure of the endodontic monoblock[1]

(2) The failure of intracoronal splinting using adhesive dentistry[2]

(3) The resurgence of partial coverage posterior restorations

(4) The recognition that molars do not benefit from placement of posts[3]

(5) Crack initiation in stress tests of endodontically treated roots[4,5]

Endodontic accesses are traditionally conservative to the occlusal/incisal tooth structure. However, with the changes that occur in restorative dentistry, this technique is unnecessarily restrictive for the operator and potentially damaging to the more critical cervical area of the tooth.

The following case is representative of a large percentage of endodontic accesses performed by general dentists and endodontists. This story is replayed each day in the United States and Canada. **Fig. 1** shows a lower first molar of a 20-year-old woman. These young teeth are dangerously hollow to begin with. By the time that both of these well-meaning dentists had finished with the tooth, the molar was nearly worthless. The most important structures were so badly compromised that the tooth was permanently crippled.

The general dentist created the first access using fissure burs and with the type of dentin removal that is the standard today (**Fig. 2**A). The tooth was then reaccessed by an internationally recognized endodontist (**Fig. 2**B, C). This model for generous removal of pericervical dentin is common in many specialty practices. Eighteen months later, the lesion on the mesial root continues to enlarge (**Fig. 3**). In the authors' practices, such a tooth does not warrant endodontic retreatment. The wholesale loss of PCD has reduced the value of this tooth to the point that, when the tooth becomes symptomatic, extraction and replacement with an implant is a better option. In fairness to their patients, dentists must change the process, or make implants a first option instead of the eventual option. The new model of endodontic access is superimposed over the tooth in **Fig. 4**.

In summary, directed dentin and enamel conservation is the best and only proven method to buttress the endodontically treated molar. No man-made material or technique can compensate for tooth structure lost in key areas of the PCD. Molar access, key to endodontic success, should also be considered as the key to restorative success and to long-term retention of the molar tooth. The primary purpose of the redesigned access is to avoid the fracturing potential of the endodontically treated molar.[7] For expediency, molar fracturing can be described as retrograde vertical root fracture; midroot vertical root fracturing; oblique root/crown fracturing; and horizontal, oblique, and vertical coronal fracturing.

A NEW MODEL FOR ENDODONTIC ACCESS

As endodontic access is deconstructed, it is crucial to understand the 5 catalyst forces that will change the future of endodontic access and coronal shaping. They are:

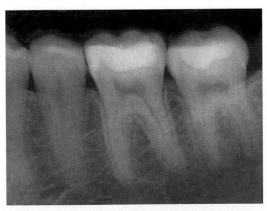

Fig. 1. Preoperative view of tooth #19 in a 20-year-old woman.

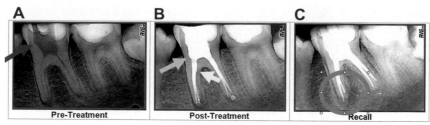

Fig. 2. (*A*) The deroofing problem. The likely bur used by the referring general dentist is a 56 carbide; one of the most popular burs in dentistry,[6] it is possibly the most iatrogenic instrument in modern medicine. Red arrow delineates the typical gouging. (*B*) Postoperative view provided by the endodontist. Blue arrow indicates the grossly excessive dentin removal of pericervical dentin (PCD). This serious gouging is typical of round bur access. Yellow arrow indicates the large canal flaring with unacceptable dentin removal (blind funneling). (*C*) Green circle highlights worsening lesion on mesial root ends.

1. Implant success rates
2. Operating microscopes and micro-endodontics
3. Biomimetic dentistry
4. Minimally invasive dentistry
5. Esthetic demands of patients.

In both of the authors' practices, the endodontic goals and armamentarium have been in a constant state of flux for nearly a decade as we have collaborated to bring the EERP continuum to maturity. The goal is to satisfy the demands of the big 5 forces for change mentioned earlier. In so doing, we have come to realize that, when cutting endodontic access, our previous needs as dentists were often in conflict with the needs of the tooth.

Table 1 presents the hierarchy of needs to maintain optimal strength, fracture resistance, and several other characteristics needed for long-term full function of the endodontically treated tooth. Banking of tooth structure is key and is age- and case-sensitive. For example, in the case of the importance of pericervical enamel, the cementoenamel junction (CEJ) is an invaluable asset in the physiologically young molar. Margins of direct and indirect restorations placed on enamel have been shown

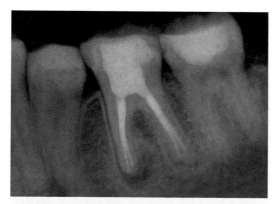

Fig. 3. Eighteen-month follow-up. Despite generous access and aggressive canal enlargement, the lesion on the mesial root continues to enlarge.

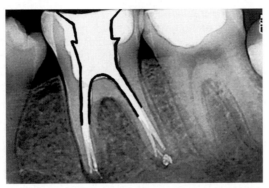

Fig. 4. A more appropriate access shape is overlayed. Partial deroofing and maintenance of a robust amount of PCD is demonstrated. A soffit that includes pulp horns on mesial and distal is depicted.

to be more caries resistant than margins on dentin. The CEJ is also the most ideal vehicle to transition the stress from crown to apex.

Three-dimensional Ferrule

Three-dimensional ferrule is the backbone of prosthetic dentistry and has historically been described as axial wall dentin covered by the axial wall of the crown or bridge abutment. Ferrules are frequently used outside of dentistry. For example, in musical instruments, a ferule is a metal band used to prevent the ends of wooden instruments from splitting. Compression fittings for attaching tubing (piping) commonly have ferrules in them. A swaged termination type for wire rope or the cap at the end of a cane or umbrella are ferrules. In pool and billiards, the portion of a cue that tops the shaft and to which the leather tip is bonded is a ferrule. In fishing, the male and female joints that join one section of a rod to the next are known as ferrules.

Research varies on the minimal vertical amount required, but the range of absolute minimums is from 1.5 mm to 2.5 mm.[8–23] The clinician must remember that buildup material, although necessary, does not count toward ferrules. A more comprehensive view of ferrules is needed, and is embodied in the term three-dimensional ferrule (3DF). There are 3 components of the new ferrule; first is the vertical component, which was

Table 1	
The hierarchy of tooth needs for posterior teeth	
Value to the Tooth	**Tissue Type**
High	PCD Undermined dentin The D^2J Axial wall DEJ Cervical enamel in the physiologic young tooth
Medium	Coronal enamel
Low	2° dentin
No value or liability	3° Dentin Undermined enamel Inflamed pulp in mature teeth Cementoenamel junction in physiologically aged tooth or in root caries–prone patient

described earlier, and is the traditional ferrule. The second component is dentin girth (thickness). The absolute minimum thickness is 1 mm; however, 2 mm is obviously a safer number. Girth becomes more important closer to the finish lines of the preparation. The thickness of the remaining dentin (the wall thickness) between the external surface of the tooth at the finish line and the endodontic access is more important apically. Further, progressing apically down onto the root surface in the endodontically treated tooth, the wall thickness can vary considerably and can become thin in places, especially if large coronal shaping or flaring was done during the endodontic treatment. Thus, axially deep finish lines on root structure can be extremely damaging to 3DF. Gutta percha is an exceptionally poor core material. The third component is total occlusal convergence (TOC) or net taper. TOC is the total draw of the 2 opposing axial walls of the prepared tooth to receive a fixed crown. A net taper or TOC of 10° requires 3 mm of vertical ferrule; a TOC of 20° requires 4 mm of vertical ferrule.[24–37] Deep chamfer marginal zones, common with modern porcelain crowns, typically have a net taper of 50° or more, and therefore many modern esthetic margins lose a millimeter or more of their original potential 3DF at the crown margin interface. In short, typical modern porcelain crown prep has less 3DF than the corresponding gold crown prep. Hence, the need for directed dentin conservation during endodontic access becomes even more crucial, and, at the same time, the volume of dentin removed in the axial direction should be questioned in the modern era of high-strength zirconia core crowns that actually allow minimal axiomarginal reduction. In certain case types and finish line designs, the degree of apical placement of the finish line can affect the ferrule quality, as mentioned earlier. Light axiomarginal reduction coupled with apically placed finish lines and a nonzero-degree emergence profile of the restoration can provide high 3DF. The concept of 3DF incorporates an interplay between these factors that, in sum, indicate the true ferrule quality.

Undermined Enamel Versus Undermined Dentin

Because undermined enamel has not been shown to be strengthened by resin restorations, it becomes a liability because of fracture potential, poor C factor, and as a physical and visual obstruction to the endodontic operator. Conversely, because dentin acts as a trimodal composite, it can be of great value to the tooth whether the undermined dentin occurs naturally, such as the soffit, or from previous restorative/endodontic treatment. It is important to clarify that the act of purposely undermining dentin for mechanical retention of restorative materials or when using round burs in endodontic access is no longer indicated in contemporary restorative and endodontic dentistry. Enamel is essentially a crystalline structure and is therefore naturally supported 100% by dentin. Dentin, by contrast, is a multilevel composite that can stand alone and acts ideally as a semirigid pipe.

PCD

PCD is the dentin near the alveolar crest. Although the apex of the root can be amputated, and the coronal third of the clinical crown removed and replaced prosthetically, the dentin near the alveolar crest is irreplaceable. This critical zone, roughly 4 mm above the crestal bone and extending 4 mm apical to the crestal bone, is important for 3 reasons: ferrule, fracturing, and dentin tubule orifice proximity from inside to out. The research is unequivocal; long-term retention of the tooth and resistance to fracturing are directly related to the amount of residual tooth structure.[9,11] The more dentin is kept, the longer the tooth is kept.

SACRIFICE VERSUS COMPROMISE

In the featured case, significant dentin was sacrificed to facilitate expedient and safe (avoidance of rotary file separation) instrumentation. No compromise was made in creating a direct pathway to the apices allowing copious irrigation and full vertical compaction of heated gutta percha, and yet the endodontic treatment was failing. Contrast that case with the tooth in **Fig. 5**. There was a significant compromise when the dentist, 20 years ago, stopped removing dentin when he or she could not find the canal systems and filled less than half of the distal root. Yet the poor endodontic result is successful, the well-preserved PCD has buttressed the tooth, and the overall case is a still a success after 20 years. The authors have seen many cases of seemingly poor endodontic results that have defied current and conventional endodontic wisdom. Without detracting from the Schilder Objectives, the case types that seem to be lacking in the long-term are those with the appearance of high-quality endodontics, namely generous endodontic access, continuous taper, and large shape, facilitating the compaction of warm gutta percha.

LOOK, GROOM, AND FOLLOW: SHAPING VERSUS MACHINING

(1) Why are Gates Glidden (GG) burs so problematic? Since the introduction of rotary files, GG burs have been used more aggressively and with more reliance on larger sizes (4, 5 and 6) to reduce binding and fracture of rotary files. Gates burs have always been considered safe because they do not end cut and are self-centering. There is a significant problem here, which is cervical self centering. Because the shank of the GG is so thin, it is difficult to steer the GG away from high-risk anatomy. As the GG straightens the coronal or high curve, it can shortcut across a fluting or furcation and weaken or even create strip perforations (**Fig. 6**). Dr Clark has abandoned, and Dr Khademi has severely curtailed, the use of GG burs in their respective practices.

(2) Why are round burs so destructive? The traditional method of initiating endodontic access is predicated on mental models that do not represent the day-to-day clinical reality presented to the clinician. Many texts shows the same round bur technique relying on tactile feedback as the round bur drops into the chamber (**Fig. 7**).

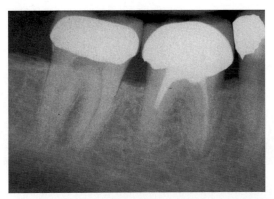

Fig. 5. Radiographically ugly but clinically successful (20 years) endodontic treatment. This case was likely done on a vital tooth. Residual PCD has buttressed this tooth to avoid fracture.

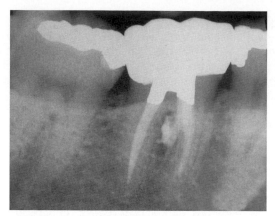

Fig. 6. Extensive coronal flaring results in extrusion of obturation material in the furcation. The furcal strip perforation is a perfect example of the dangers of blind funneling with GG burs.

These kinds of images, so frequently shown in dental school, textbooks, and lectures, are predicated on mental models based on occlusal decay in children. If the pulp chamber is sufficiently large, then a round bur can truly drop in to the pulp chamber, as shown in **Fig. 8**, with a #6 round bur superimposed on the lower molar of an 11-year-old child.

The reality of day-to-day clinical practice is far removed from this, and these deeply ingrained mental models are a setup for occult iatrogenic trauma. More realistically,

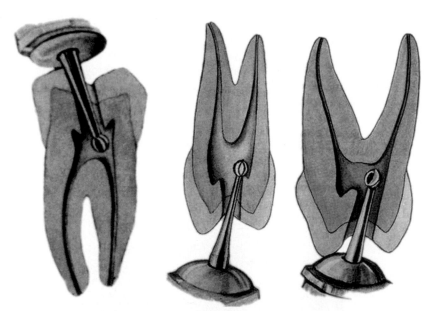

Fig. 7. Texts frequently show the same round bur technique relying on tactile feedback as the round bur drops into the chamber. (*From* Ingle JI, Beveridge EE. Endodontics. 2nd edition. Lea and Febiger; 1976. p. 132 (plate XII), 148 (plate XX), 157 (plate XXIV); with permission.)

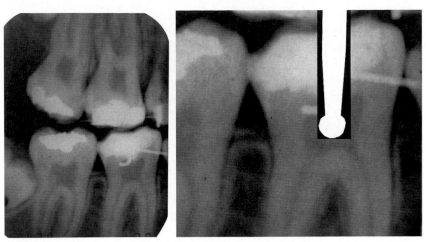

Fig. 8. If the pulp chamber is sufficiently large, then a round bur can drop in to the pulp chamber, as shown here with a #6 round bur superimposed on the lower molar of this 11-year-old child.

the case shown in **Fig. 9** is more representative of the spectrum of cases typically presenting for endodontic treatment. Clearly, trying to drop a round bur into the scant or nonexistent chamber is not going to lead to the desired outcome even for a skilled clinician. Instead, the size of the burs relative to the chambers, the omnidirectional cutting blades (which side cut aggressively), and chatter common with this bur design are much more likely to lead to the kinds of outcomes seen in **Figs. 2** and **3**.

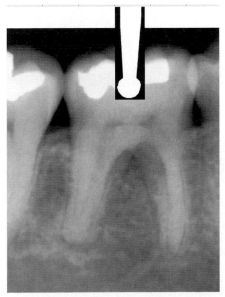

Fig. 9. The case shown here is more representative of the spectrum of cases typically presenting for endodontic treatment. Trying to drop a round bur into the scant or nonexistent chamber is not going to lead to the desired outcome even for a skilled clinician.

So although round burs are destructive because they contribute to, or exacerbate, these problems, it is really the tactile-based mental models predicated on these kinds of drawings showing round burs dropping into the pulp that are the ultimate problem. Care and magnification can compensate, but only to a degree (**Fig. 10**).

(3) Why is complete deroofing so dangerous? When the authors first began to maintain a soffit, which is a small piece of roof around the entire coronal portion of the pulp chamber, it seemed sloppy and contradicted the compulsive nature of traditional dentistry that has made complete deroofing a mark of a thorough clinician. The pulp seemed difficult to remove under the tiny eve and the removal of sealer and gutta percha was equally difficult. It just seemed wrong. Today it makes perfect sense; cleanup is easier and the authors take pride in this important advance in minimally invasive access. It is a perfect example of banked tooth structure. However, it is the attempts at removing the soffit that are far more damaging to the surrounding PCD. The idea that a round bur can be dropped below this soffit and drawn coronally to unroof the chamber is predicated on large pulp chambers and exceptional hand skills. Clinically, it is impossible. Attempting to remove the pulp chamber roof does not accomplish any real endodontic objective, and invariably gouges the walls that are responsible for long-term survival of the tooth. The primary reason to maintain the soffit is to avoid the collateral damage that usually occurs, namely the gouging of the lateral walls. Research will certainly need to be done to validate the strength attributes of the roof strut or soffit. However, in the absence of a compelling

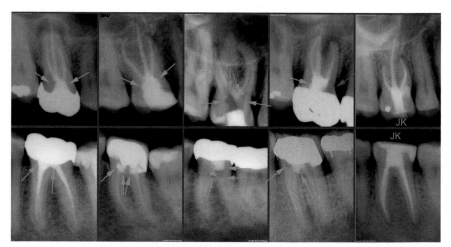

Fig. 10. Blue arrows indicate gouges. Red arrows indicate perforations. Essentially, all previously accessed molars were gouged to some degree. The first upper and lower molar cases show what many might consider acceptable access extension, and were obviously cut with round burs. Both are gouged. The third upper and lower cases have frighteningly thin pulpal floors with blushing dentin. The upper fourth case is deceptive in that it is perforated, whereas the worse-looking lower case is not, but the pulpal floor is thin. The last upper molar case (which has a class V resorption repair) shows what is possible with practice, microscope level magnification, an assistant, and the right instruments. The lower molar shows the type of access that should be routinely achievable with high-powered loupes and the right instruments. (JK indicates that the case was done by John Khademi with adherence to the modern model of directed dentin conservation.)

reason to remove dentin, our default position should always be conservative. This 360° soffit or roof-wall interface can also be compared with the metal ring that stabilizes a wooden barrel. Inference to the second moment of inertia in structural engineering deserves analysis. The second potential benefit, as described earlier, is embodied in the physics model of the second moment of inertia. An ideal example of second moment of inertia is the I beam. The second moment or furthest point of the I portion away from the center of the beam, or centroid, determines the resistance to bending. Maintaining dentin as it rounds a corner places it far from the cervical area, which is often where fracturing initiates in the endodontically accessed molar. More important than the soffit itself, however, is the preservation of axial wall dentin near the soffit.

Presuming one could drop into the pulp chamber in the way described earlier (see **Fig. 7**), the chamber roof is now to be removed by scooping it up and away with a round carbide. A two-dimensional drawing with the small size of the bur and chamber roof overhanging a large pulp chamber makes this seem like a reasonable proposition. The chamber walls are always drawn flat even though they are cut by a round bur.

In practice, it is impossible to cut flat walls in 3 dimensions with a round instrument. The chamber is not unroofed in some areas, leaving pulpal and necrotic debris with no specific subsequent step to address the debris, yet the walls are overextended and gouged in other areas. Further, the internal radius of curvature at many of the pulp chamber line angles is simply too small for all but the smallest of round burs.

In the final analysis, round burs point cut in an endodontic access application, whereas what is needed is planing. What is needed is a new set of mental models based on vision, and a new set of instruments reflective of the task at hand and the desired shaping outcomes. The new vision-based mental model is *Look, Groom, Follow*. The new burs are all round-ended tapers (**Fig. 11**).

It is appropriate to provide updated cavosurface outlines and cross-sectional illustrations for initial access for the maxillary and mandibular molars (**Table 2**).

CAVOSURFACE AND CROSS-SECTIONAL ILLUSTRATIONS FOR MAXILLARY MOLAR ACCESS

Traditional textbooks devote considerable length and effort on drawing access outline forms that are done on restoration-free, caries-free teeth. The authors hesitate to provide access outline drawings as there are so many variables that enter into the formula on real clinical cases. Within this context, the authors provide these drawings as a guideline for accessing full coverage gold or porcelain for cases in which the underlying restorative materials, the presence or absence of decay, and the locations of sound dentin cannot be ascertained. When in doubt, a larger outline form through the restorative should be cut, but only to the level at which dentin is encountered. Then, the access should be vision based, cuing from the color map and the presence of any PTRs that can be identified. This method is a stepped access, in which an intentionally over-enlarged access is made through the cavosurface of a restored tooth (typically a crowned tooth) to the level at which dentin is encountered, then the access steps in to the size of the pulp chamber outline.

The occlusal view drawing shows an inner outline form in black, requiring the most sophistication in skill and magnification. Suggested extensions for clinicians at different points along the experience/magnification curve in blue and green show extension and enlargement, primarily toward the mesial and buccal. These should be primarily interpreted as the direction to strategically extend the access based on

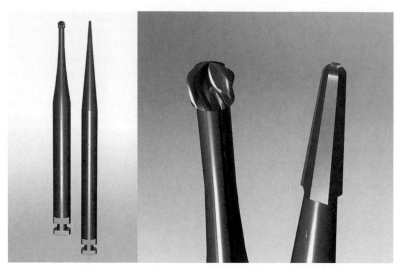

Fig. 11. Comparison of the CK endodontic access bur with the corresponding round bur. The tip size of these burs is less than half as wide as the corresponding round bur. One of the prototype CK endodontic access burs (*right*) is shown and contrasted with the corresponding surgical length round bur (*left*). These burs, designed by Drs Clark and Khademi, will be available from SS White Burs, Inc.

experience/magnification and case difficulty as opposed to absolute outline forms. The angles of entry into the canal system are unlikely to be perpendicular to the occlusal surface. The access rarely needs to be significantly extended to the distal or palatal, as the angle of entry to the palatal canal is out to the mesio-buccal (MB) (**Fig. 12**), and the distal is toward the mesio-palatal (MP) (**Fig. 13**). The MB and MB2 angles of entry are generally from the distal, and can also be from the palatal (**Figs. 14** and **15**).

Table 2
The 6 types of molar cavosurface and chamber access

Restorative Case Type	Cavosurface Angle (To Occlusal Table)
Nonmutilated molar to receive bonded indirect onlay or composite onlay	1 mm of anatomic flattening (2 mm cusp tip flattening); then 45° angle of penetration until reaching the dentinal map (Fig. 20)
Nonmutilated molar to receive full crown	1.5 mm of anatomic flattening (2.5 mm cusp tip flattening); then 45° angle of penetration until reaching the dentin map
Mutilated molar to receive full crown	2–3 mm of flattening
Gold crown to be retained	80° angle of penetration until reaching the dentin map
PFM crown to be retained	45° angle of penetration through the crown until reaching the dentin map
Zirconia based porcelain crown* to be maintained	70–90° angle of penetration until reaching the dentin map

* As of date of publish, most zirconia based crowns including Lava tm and Procera tm have non etchable cores and non etchable stacked porcelains.

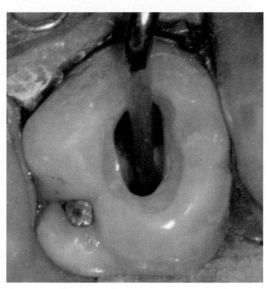

Fig. 12. The angle of entry to the palatal canal is out to the MB.

An access extension or modification that is frequently needed is the fluting or notching of the mesial wall in the area of the MB2. This requirement is due to the pattern of calcification that often places the angle of entry to the MB2 at an untenable distal angle. This notching can be performed in dentin with a BUC-1 ultrasonic tip, and, if need be, extended into restorative using an LAAxxess nipple-tipped diamond. This case (**Fig. 16**) shows a preliminary access with a slight amount of fluting (**Fig. 17**). A closeup shows the finished fluting in the prepared case, and the overall sizes of the access through the porcelain fused to metal (PFM) (crown) and the dentin (**Figs. 18**

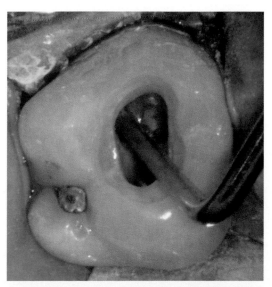

Fig. 13. The angle of entry to the distal canal is out to the MP.

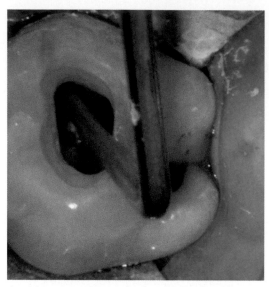

Fig. 14. The MB angles of entry are generally from the distal side.

and **19**). A frequent criticism of the techniques demonstrated here is that these more precise shapes preclude the discovery of coronal points of negotiation (PONs), and deep anatomy, and preclude the development of condensation hydraulics. The authors have not found this to be the case. In this case with an apparent confluent MB/MB2, precurved files were introduced with intent on the palatal aspect of the MB2, which often contains a deep split. The wire radiograph shows the 2 larger files, 1 in the MB orifice and 1 in the MB2 orifice joining, and a smaller file, also in the MB2

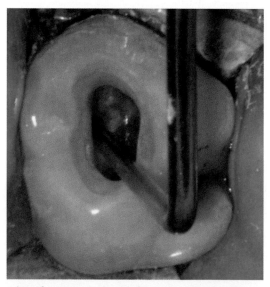

Fig. 15. The MB2 angles of entry can also be from the palatal side.

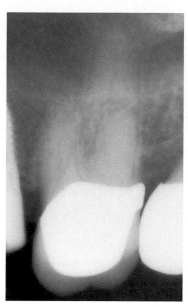

Fig. 16. Preoperative condition.

orifice branching deep to a separate portal of exit (**Fig. 20**). The completed case is shown in **Fig. 21**.

As discussed earlier, these should be interpreted more as guides on how and where to extend, rather than as absolute extension guidelines. The first 2 buccal views show a large pulp chamber (**Fig. 22**), and a raw Clark/Khademi (CK)-style access with small

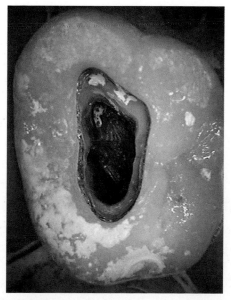

Fig. 17. Initial access, slight fluting.

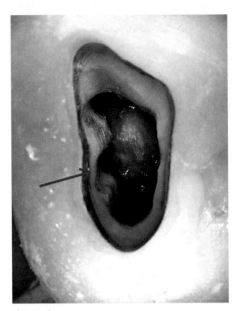

Fig. 18. Closeup fluting (*arrow*).

soffits of chamber roof left to be debrided later (**Fig. 23**). The next buccal view is an overlay of the CK-style access, a more traditional occlusally divergent access, and an access taken from a recent text showing fairly parallel walls, but grossly overextended cervically (**Fig. 24**). The second set of overlays shows the CK-style access with blue and green extensions, with cavosurface finish lines appropriate for a bonded

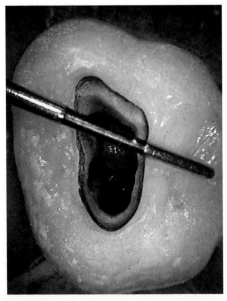

Fig. 19. Access with probe.

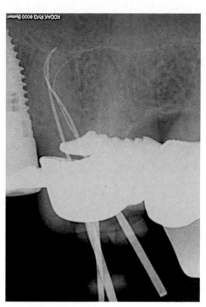

Fig. 20. Working radiograph.

substrate with a bonded restorative, which are described later (**Fig. 25**). The mesial view shows the various extensions, again emphasizing the directions to extend as opposed to exact amounts and locations (**Fig. 26**). The extension is not balanced equally between buccal and palatal, but favors the buccal.

The guiding principles and strategy on access and access extension should recognize the hierarchy of tooth needs listed in **Table 1**. Restorative materials should almost

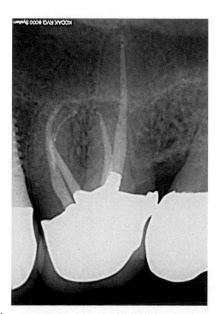

Fig. 21. Final radiograph.

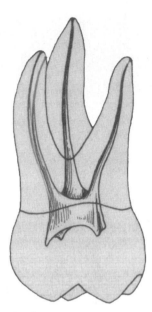

Fig. 22. Buccal view with normal pulp.

always be sacrificed before tooth structure. More occlusal tooth structure should be sacrificed for more cervical tooth structure. The key pericerivcal tooth structure should remain as untouched as possible.

Final cavosurface outline extension at the finish appointment (which may be the start appointment on a 1-step case) hinges on the existing restorative, and the restorative plan. If abundant highly bondable substrate such as etchable porcelain or

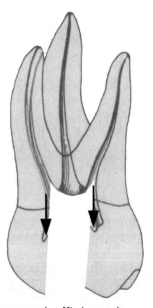

Fig. 23. Buccal view with CK access and soffit (*arrows*).

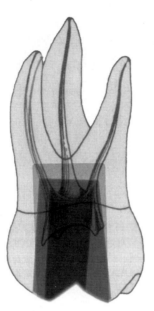

Fig. 24. Buccal view with access overlays.

enamel is available, and a bondable restorative material such as a heavily filled composite resin is planned, the cavosurface should be Cala Lillied (**Fig. 27**), or generously beveled on those areas. If the bondability of the substrate is of low, or a bond cannot be established between the substrate and restorative material, a butt joint or 70 to 90° interface at the cavosurface should be the objective. On multiple visit cases in which an unbonded temporary restoration is placed, the cavosurface should be maintained at 70 to 90° until the completion visit.

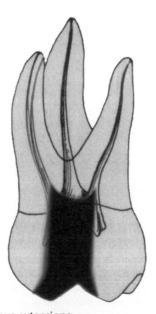

Fig. 25. Buccal view with various extensions.

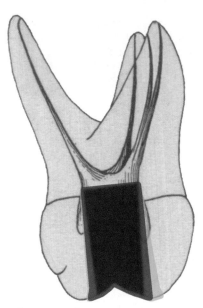

Fig. 26. Mesial view with various extensions.

CAVOSURFACE AND CROSS-SECTIONAL ILLUSTRATIONS FOR MANDIBULAR MOLAR ACCESS

These illustrations are consistent with the style of access demonstrated in the maxillary molar section earlier (generously flared and flattened when appropriate in the coronal third of the tooth, then conservative in the middle and apical portion of the coronal portion of the tooth).

The first step in contemporary molar access in the noncrowned tooth is flattening. It is a step that is ignored or overdone in most practices.

GUIDELINES FOR TREATMENT DECISIONS

There have been some consistent patterns in what the authors have observed in their practices with the long-term successful cases. These observations are important for

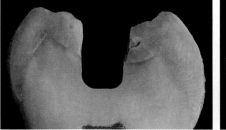 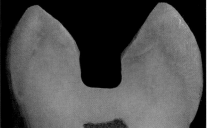

Fig. 27. Traditional parallel-sided access (*left*), compared with the Cala Lilly enamel preparation (*right*). (*Left*) Unfavorable C factor and poor enamel rod engagement are typically present when removing old amalgam or composite restorations or with traditional endodontic access of 90° to the occlusal table. (*Right*) The enamel is cut back at 45° with the Cala Lilly shape. This modified preparation will now allow engagement of nearly the entire occlusal surface.

2 reasons: (1) they can serve to direct how virgin endo/restorative cases planned for treatment are managed; (2) they can help the endodontist quickly decide whether retreating failing prior treatment is even worth investigating. Although it would be advantageous for the treating clinician to have objective randomized clinical trials (RCTs) on the factors related to long-term endodontic success, there is a dearth of RCTs of longer than 20 years to guide the clinician with the real variables related to long-term success. The authors are, however, able to observe the cases presenting to their practices. These observations contradict contemporary endodontic thinking, yet, when put to the test, remain essentially unchallenged. They are certain to cause controversy in the endodontic community:

(1) Long-term, that is, 20- to 40-year, success of the endodontically treated tooth has little to do with what would be traditionally characterized as the quality of the endodontic result.
(2) Preservation of dentin trumps quality endodontics when evaluated over a time frame of 20 to 40 years.

The Three Strikes Rule

In endodontically treated cases from 20 to 40 years ago, the authors have observed consistently that these teeth are violated in less than 3 ways. The cases that truly go the distance have damage in 2 or less of the following clinically controllable variables:

(1) Excessive axial reduction (consistent with PFM or all-porcelain restorations)
(2) Gouged endodontic access
(3) Large and arbitrarily round endodontic shape.

   The authors would contend that teeth that are violated in 3 or more ways simply do not go the distance. All 3 of these violations are insults to the PCD, and if all 3 are present, the loss of PCD is irreparable and the tooth is permanently compromised or destroyed. When the clinician is evaluating a case for possible treatment, it is far more advantageous and expedient to evaluate the restorative aspects of the case first. One should ask: "Presuming successful endodontic treatment, what is left to work with?" For instance, if the distal half of the tooth is severely decayed, but the patient has adequate opening, the access can be distalized, directing dentin conservation to the mesial half of the tooth, leaving the opportunity for enough 3DF.
   With retreatment cases, the rationale is the same, and the question to ask, before even considering the endodontic issues, is: "How many ways has this tooth been violated?" If the tooth has been violated 2 or more ways (ie, 3 strikes), it is exceptionally unlikely that a long-term result can be delivered to the patient with even the most exceptional endodontic care.

GLOSSARY OF TERMS FOR CONTEMPORARY MOLAR ENDODONTIC ACCESS

   • The endodontic-endorestorative-prosthodontic (EERP) continuum

   The EERP is a restoratively driven view of the endodontics as simply a servant to the restoration and preservation of the tooth, concurrent with a complete integration of endodontic design as part of an interlocking series of components. From crown to apex an outside fortress of fracture resistance, and from inside to outside a set of firewalls for leakage prevention. Biomimetics and minimally invasive dentistry are guiding principles. Each component must compliment, not compromise, the other components. If at any point in the diagnosis, access, endodontic shaping, or obturation a critical compromise is discovered, the ethical directive demands that extraction and implant placement must be considered in lieu of continuation of the attempt to retain the tooth.

- Three-dimensional ferrule (3DF)

3DF is an evaluation of the available dentin that will buttress the crown. The 3 components are dentin height, dentin girth (dentin thickness), and TOC (total draw of the opposing axial walls; buccal-lingual and mesial-distal).

- Pericervical dentin (PCD)

PCD is defined as the dentin near the alveolar crest. This critical zone, roughly 4 mm coronal to the crestal bone and extending 4 mm apical to crestal bone, is crucial to transferring load from the occlusal table to the root, and much of the PCD is irreplaceable.

- Banked tooth structure

The approach of banking of tooth structure in restorative dentistry dictates that whenever possible, more tooth structure should be left in place than is needed for the procedure at hand. It may involve a less expedient, but more conservative, approach. This banked tooth structure may serve as a valuable future asset in the advent of unforeseen future trauma or disease, coupled with the reality that a tooth will need to last for decades and potentially be restored and then rerestored in the patient's lifetime.

- *The inverse funnel*

An undesirable endodontic access shape in which the size of the access becomes wider as it progresses deeper into the tooth. It is a common occurrence when constricted cavosurface access opening size is paired with round bur use. It is exacerbated when advanced magnification is not used during tooth cutting.

- *Blind tunneling*

Blind tunneling is another undesirable endodontic access approach and shape that creates a parallel sided access when performed without advanced magnification, relying on tactile feedback rather than on microscopic visualization and following the dentinal maps of primary, secondary, and tertiary dentin and microscopic traces of residual pulp tissue. Typically performed with round burs.

- *Blind funneling*

Blind funneling is another undesirable access shape, common in generalist and endodontic specialist practices. This popular practice obliterates significant tooth structure to facilitate rapid and safe (avoidance of file separation) machining of the roots with rotary files.

- Filling and caries leveraged access
- Partial deroofing
- Soffit
- Stepped access
- Secondary dentin (2° dentin)

- Tertiary dentin (3° dentin)
- Biomimetic endodontic shaping (BES)
- *Arbitrary round shaping (ARS)*
- The dentinal map
- The dentinoenamel junction (DEJ)
- The junction of primary and secondary dentin (D^2J)
- The junction of primary and tertiary dentin (D^3J)
- Pulp tissue remnants (PTRs)
- The Cala Lilly

Fig. 27 highlights the creation of the Cala Lilly cavity shape. The Cala Lilly is a flower and is the new model for composite preparations.

- Points of negotiation (PONs)

PONs are statistically predictable anatomic areas that may serve as starting points during the access portion of endodontic therapy.

Italicized points indicate an undesirable outcome or technique.

ACKNOWLEDGMENTS

Dr Clark would like to thank Dr Jihyon Kim, Dr Eric Herbransen and Dr Marc Balson, for their input and unwavering support.

REFERENCES

1. Tay FR, Pashley DH. Monoblocks in root canals: a hypothetical or a tangible goal. J Endod 2007;33(4):391–8.
2. Wahl MJ, Schmitt MM, Overton DA, et al. Prevalence of cusp fractures in teeth restored with amalgam and with resin-based composite. J Am Dent Assoc 2004;135:1127–32.
3. Schwartz RS, Robbins JW. Post placement and restoration of endodontically treated teeth: a literature review. J Endod 2004;30(5):289–301.
4. Lirtchirakarn V. Patterns of vertical root fractures: factors affecting stress distribution in the root canal. J Endod 2003;29:523–8.
5. Tamse A. An evaluation of endodontically treated vertically fractured teeth. J Endod 1999;25:506–8.
6. Miles B. Sales data. New Jersey: SS White Bur Inc; 2008.
7. Tan PL, Aquilino SA, Gratton DG, et al. In vitro fracture resistance of endodontically treated central incisors with varying ferrule heights and configurations. J Prosthet Dent 2005;93(4):331–6.
8. Sahafi A, Peutzfeldt A, Ravnholt G, et al. Resistance to cyclic loading of teeth restored with posts. Clin Oral Investig 2005;9(2):84–90.
9. Kutesa-Mutebi A, Osman YI. Effect of the ferrule on fracture resistance of teeth restored with prefabricated posts and composite cores. Afr Health Sci 2004; 4(2):131–5.
10. Akkayan B. An in vitro study evaluating the effect of ferrule length on fracture resistance of endodontically treated teeth restored with fiber-reinforced and zirconia dowel systems. J Prosthet Dent 2004;92(2):155–62.
11. Goto Y, Nicholls JI, Phillips KM, et al. Fatigue resistance of endodontically treated teeth restored with three dowel-and-core systems. J Prosthet Dent 2005;93(1): 45–50.

12. Ng CC, al-Bayat MI, Dumbrigue HB, et al. Effect of no ferrule on failure of teeth restored with bonded posts and cores. Gen Dent 2004;52(2):143–6.
13. Smidt A, Venezia E. The use of an existing cast post and core as an anchor for extrusive movement. Int J Prosthodont 2003;16(3):225–8.
14. Pierrisnard L, Bohin F, Renault P, et al. Corono-radicular reconstruction of pulp-less teeth: a mechanical study using finite element analysis. J Prosthet Dent 2002;88(4):442–8.
15. Stankiewicz NR, Wilson PR. The ferrule effect: a literature review. Int Endod J 2002;35(7):575–81. Review.
16. Hsu YB, Nicholls JI, Phillips KM, et al. Effect of core bonding on fatigue failure of compromised teeth. Int J Prosthodont 2002;15(2):175–8.
17. Lenchner NH. Considering the "ferrule effect". Pract Proced Aesthet Dent 2001; 13(2):102.
18. al-Hazaimeh N, Gutteridge DL. An in vitro study into the effect of the ferrule preparation on the fracture resistance of crowned teeth incorporating prefabricated post and composite core restorations. Int Endod J 2001;34(1):40–6.
19. Gegauff AG. Effect of crown lengthening and ferrule placement on static load failure of cemented cast post-cores and crowns. J Prosthet Dent 2000;84(2):169–79.
20. Morgano SM, Brackett SE. Foundation restorations in fixed prosthodontics: current knowledge and future needs [review]. J Prosthet Dent 1999;82(6):643–57.
21. Hunter AJ, Hunter AR. The treatment of endodontically treated teeth. Curr Opin Dent 1991;1(2):199–205. Review.
22. Loney RW, Kotowicz WE, McDowell GC. Three-dimensional photoelastic stress analysis of the ferrule effect in cast post and cores. J Prosthet Dent 1990;63(5): 506–12.
23. Jorgensen KD. The relationship between retention and convergence angle in cemented veneer crowns. Acta Odontol Scand 1955;13:35–40.
24. Wilson AH, Chan DC. The relationship between preparation convergence and retention of extracoronal retainers. J Prosthodont 1994;3:74–8.
25. Smith CT, Gary JJ, Conkin JE, et al. Effective taper criterion for the full veneer crown preparation in preclinical prosthondontics. J Prosthodont 1999;8:196–200.
26. Noonan JE Jr, Goldfogel MH. Convergence of the axial walls of full veneer crown preparations in a dental school environment. J Prosthet Dent 1991;66:706–8.
27. Ohm E, Silness J. The convergence angle in teeth prepared for artificial crowns. J Oral Rehabil 1978;5:371–5.
28. Annerstedt A, Engstrom U, Hansson A, et al. Axial wall convergence of full veneer crown preparations. Documented for dental students and general practitioners. Acta Odontal Scand 1996;54:109–12.
29. Lempoel PJ, Snoek PA, van't Hof M, et al. [The convergence angel of crown preparations with clinically satisfactory retention]. Ned Tijdschr Tandheelkd 1993;100: 336–8 [in Dutch].
30. Mou SH, Chai T, Wang JS, et al. Influence of different convergence angles and tooth preparation heights on the internal adaptation of Cerec crowns. J Prosthet Dent 2002;87:248–55.
31. Dodge WW, Weed RM, Baez RJ, et al. The effect of convergence angle on retention and resistance form. Quintessence Int 1985;16:191–4.
32. Shillingburg HT, Hobo S, Whitset LD, et al. Fundamentals of fixed prosthodontics. 3rd edition. Chicago: Quintessence; 1997.
33. Wiskott HW, Nicholls JI, Belser UC. The relationship between abutment taper and resistance of cemented crowns to dynamic loading. Int J Prosthodont 1996;9: 117–39.

34. Trier AC, Parker MH, Cameron SM, et al. Evaluation of resistance form of dislodged crowns and retainers. J Prosthet Dent 1998;80:405–9.
35. Maxwell AW, Blank LW, Pelleu GB Jr. Effect of crown preparation height on the retention and resistance of gold castings. Gen Dent 1990;38:200–2.
36. Park MH, Calverley MJ, Gardner FM, et al. New guidelines for preparation taper. J Prosthodont 1993;2:61–6.
37. Woolsey GD, Matich JA. The effect of axial grooves on the resistance form of cast restorations. J Am Dent Assoc 1978;97:978–80.

Case Studies in Modern Molar Endodontic Access and Directed Dentin Conservation

David Clark, DDS[a],*, John A. Khademi, DDS, MS[b]

KEYWORDS

• Maxillary • Composite • Pulp horn • Molar

The following case studies provide insight into the integration of the principles set forward in the preceding article. Each case is evaluated first on the endorestorative principles that form the basis of the modern endo-endorestorative–prosthodontic continuum. Endorestorative needs should, whenever possible, trump previous notions of endodontic needs.

Case 1 is provided by Dr Clark, and cases 2 to 6 are provided by Dr Khademi. Dr Clark's provides a stark contrast between the old and new models of endodontic access and shaping. Dr Clark then risks avoiding postplacement but also avoids the mutilating effects of a full crown by instead providing a minimally invasive restorative technique using direct composite to permanently splint the tooth for ideal function.

Case 2 shows the possibilities in a maxillary molar when an emphasis is made on banking of coronal and pericervical dentin (PCD). The conscientious preservation of tooth structure during access and endodontic shaping allows a second, and possibly third, prosthesis (crown) during the patient's lifetime.

Case 3 is an ideal study of the realities of day to day endodontic access. This thought provoking access teaches that the authors are not accessing a crown, but accessing the root through the crown. This tipped and rotated maxillary molar; is also mutilated and coronally altered with a PFM crown creating a mirage that could easily lead to gouging and even perforation unless the operator follows the disciplined approach outlined in the text.

Case 4 is an access through another PFM crown. The importance of proper accessing through full crowns should not be underestimated, as the pulpal death rate from a full crown procedure has been documented in some studies to be well over 20%.

[a] 3402 South 38th Street, Tacoma, WA 98409, USA
[b] 2277 West 2nd Avenue, Durango, CO 81301-4658, USA
* Corresponding author.
E-mail address: drclark@microscopedentistry.com

Dent Clin N Am 54 (2010) 275–289
doi:10.1016/j.cden.2010.01.003
0011-8532/10/$ – see front matter © 2010 Elsevier Inc. All rights reserved.

dental.theclinics.com

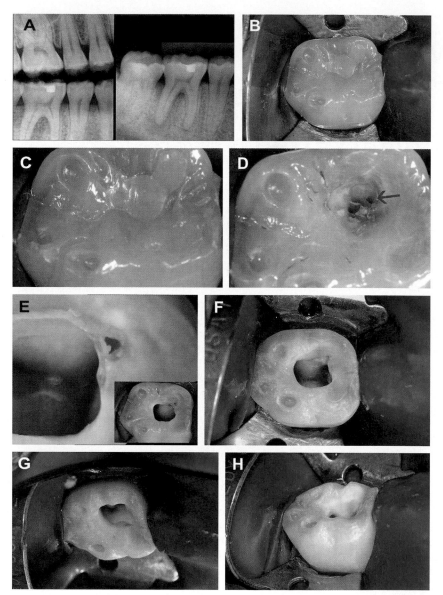

Fig. 1. (*A–T*) Case 1, the nonmutilated lower first molar to receive a direct composite onlay.

This maxillary first molar demonstrates 6 canal systems, three in the mesio-buccal root alone. The aggressive lateral removal of PCD to access the MB-2 canal system is the only such example shown in the chapter, and is warranted because the enormous amount of dentin present in this unique zone and the dangers associated with the extremely high curve of the MB-2.

Case 5 is a hallmark of both non traditional and carefully individualized access. It is the best example of capitulation to the hierarchy of tooth needs of all the cases presented in the chapter.

Case 6 demonstrates the futility of the round bur in endodontic access. The roof of the calcified lower molar chamber is sawed off and broken loose with a tapering

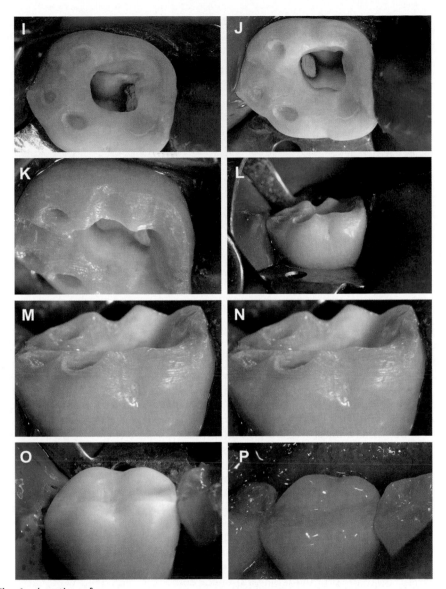

Fig. 1. (*continued*)

diamond or carbide followed by a prying excavator, not blindly and clumsily burrowed into with a round bur.

The reader is encouraged to visit and revisit these cases to fully absorb the anatomic and restorative techniques that are simultaneously presented in this very unique method of case presentation.

CASE 1: THE NONMUTILATED LOWER FIRST MOLAR TO RECEIVE A DIRECT COMPOSITE ONLAY

The preoperative bitewing (**Fig. 1**A) depicts what seems to be a very shallow and minimally invasive class I composite, but the periapical radiograph reveals periapical

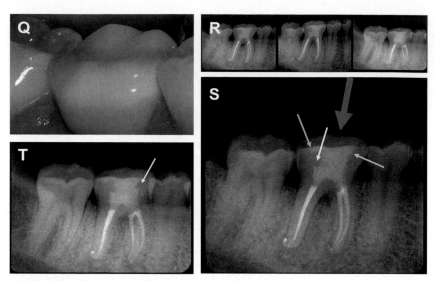

Fig. 1. (*continued*)

infections, indicating that the pulp must have been exposed at the time of treatment. **Fig. 1**B shows a low-magnification view of the occlusal surface of tooth No. 30. **Fig. 1**C is a high-magnification view (×8) of the occlusal surface. The composite restoration seems to be minimally invasive and relatively well sealed. **Fig. 1**D shows that as a saucer-shaped cut is made to explore the composite restoration and to begin endodontic access, the bur is angled at 45° instead of being parallel to the long axis of the tooth. There was a lack of bond and carious invasion along the wall of the composite restoration. This is an extremely common problem for the parallel-sided composite preparations of today. Previously exposed mesiolingual (ML) pulp horn is highlighted with red arrow.

Fig. 1E shows a ×24 magnification view, revealing that there is no such thing as a small pulp exposure. The pulp chamber is now accessed by leveraging into the chamber through the filling and caries base of operation. A small sacrifice of additional enamel with a 45° enamel wall would have allowed an ideal restorative seal and could have aided the clinician to avoid burrowing into and subsequently failing to recognize the pulp horn. Similarly, a 45° opening through the enamel for endodontic access allows better visualization, better enamel engagement, improved C factor, and improved ability to splint the tooth with direct composite. **Fig. 1**F–J were captured with a traditional flash (as opposed to coaxial microscopic light) to demonstrate the good access and lighting that is possible when delicate flattening and a 45° initial penetration is performed. In spite of what initially seems to be an insufficient cervical enlargement of the chamber, the cavosurface preparation allows reasonable endodontic access and light while maintaining generous cervical dentin.

Multiple angles of the anatomic shortening of the corona of the tooth are shown in **Fig. 1**K, L. As discussed later, it is of utmost importance to retain large islands of enamel on the occlusal of the molar tooth to avoid overreliance on dentin bonding to retain the bonded onlay. A clearance range of 1 to 2 mm is adequate for proper strength of modern microfilled composites. The rough polish of the composite onlay is demonstrated in **Fig. 1**O. **Fig. 1**P, Q shows the final polish after occlusal adjustment. Dr Clark is confident that the patient would enjoy a 10- to 20-year service from the restoration. It is the least invasive of all of the options required to splint the endodontically treated molar.

Three differently angled radiographs of the finished cusp tip-to-apex endodontic treatment are shown in **Fig. 1R. Fig. 1S** shows the first angled radiograph. The green arrow marks the 1.25-mm cuspal coverage, whereas the yellow arrow marks the soffit of dentin that was maintained and the filled pulp horn. The blue arrow marks the 45° cut through the enamel, and the large red arrow marks the mesialized access angle, which is situationally correct because the caries and filling material were encountered in the mesial portion of the tooth—a perfect example of the filling- and caries-leveraged access.

Fig. 1T shows the second angled radiograph with the yellow arrow marking the mesial soffit. After a 6-week calcium hydroxide treatment, there was an improvement (decrease) in the size of the radiographic lesions, especially the distal ones. The series of photographs, **Fig. 1A–Q**, shows an ideal bucco-occlusal-lingual composite onlay preparation, composite placement, matte finish, and final finish after occlusion was adjusted.

The chamber was carefully layered with flowable composite (Filtek Supreme Flow A-1; 3M, St Paul, MN, USA), mitigating the difficult C-factor problems by allowing the layers (2-mm increments) to touch only 1 or 2 cavity walls and never all the 4 walls at once. The cusps were built carefully with paste composite (Filtek Supreme Plus A-1 body [3M] was used with patient consent to show contrast for the photographs for a bright result) to avoid cross tooth contact during photo-polymerization of the composite. The distobuccal (DB) and distal cusps were built together with the ML cusp then photo polymerized. Then the distolingual (DL) cusp was built with the mesiobuccal (MB) cusp then photo polymerized. Although a discussion of restoratives is beyond the scope of this article, the modern version of endodontic access is constantly mindful of the restorative needs of the tooth, and that is why this brief synopsis on the composite onlay is included, to demonstrate how the ideal access leads to the ideal restoration.

CASE 2

This case demonstrates the access and restorative technique for an upper molar deemed suitable for final restoration with a bonded porcelain onlay or a composite onlay (**Fig. 2A, B**). The initial presentation of the case was a somewhat calcified molar with some slight cracking and ditching of the enamel, coincident with the natural anatomic grooves. The cusps were flattened 2 mm with wheel diamond, and the central groove area was slightly flattened. This was planned to be a 2-step procedure, which presents temporization issues if a 45° initial penetration is made, because nonbonded materials generally need to be at a 90° angle. Thus, the calla lily–shaped portion of the access is delayed until the final restorative is placed. After removing the amalgam, a residual pulp horn is noted at the MB (**Fig. 2C**). The chamber is troughed out as previously described, using Clark/Khademi (CK) burs (SS White burs Inc, NJ, USA) or ultrasonics, and 3 initial point of negotiations (PONs) are located, and an initial trough for the MB2 is made using a CK bur (**Fig. 2D**). If the opening permits, the notching for access to the MB2 can be reduced, or as in this case, nearly eliminated (**Fig. 2E**). Calcium hydroxide is placed, Cavit (3M, St Paul, MN, USA) is placed deeply with no sponge or cotton pellet, and 2–3-mm unbonded flowable composite veneer is placed over the Cavit (**Fig. 2F**). At the second visit, the procedure is completed, the chamber is cleaned up, and the calla lily portion of the access is completed (**Fig. 2G**). Separate dentin- and enamel-bonding steps are then performed (**Fig. 2H**). A small amount of flowable composite is placed over the gutta-percha and worked

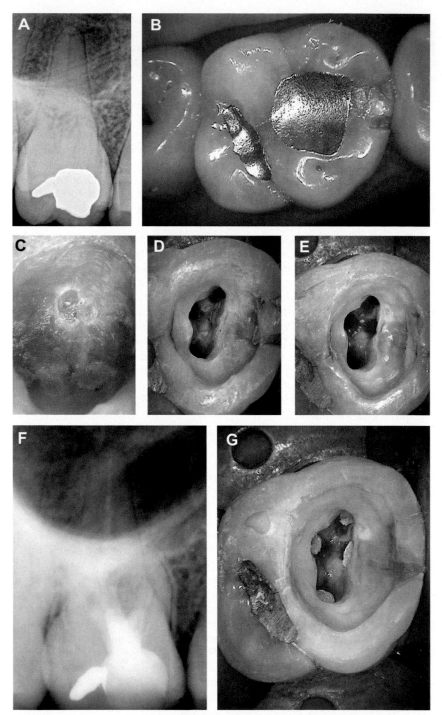

Fig. 2. (A–O) Case 2, the access and restorative technique for an upper molar deemed suitable for final restoration with a bonded porcelain onlay or composite onlay restoration.

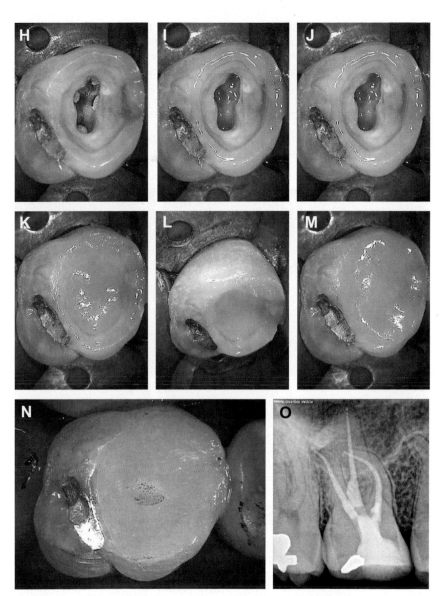

Fig. 2. (continued)

into the enamel periphery and cured (**Fig. 2**I). PhotoCore (Kuraray America, Inc, New York, NY, USA) is placed in the cervical portion of the access and cured (**Fig. 2**J). A second increment of PhotoCore is placed with the objective of creating a nearly C-factor–1 bowl for the final increment of PhotoCore (**Fig. 2**K); **Fig. 2**L shows a different view of the bowl configuration of the final increment of PhotoCore. The final increment of PhotoCore is placed and brushed to the enamel periphery (**Fig. 2**M). Occlusion is adjusted to completely eliminate any excursive contacts. Ideal occlusion in this type of case is a light single centric stop on restorative (**Fig. 2**N). The final radiograph shows a narrow "waist" to the access, which constricts from the level of the alveolar crest until it steps out to where the original amalgam was and then reflares again for maximal enamel engagement at the cavosurface (**Fig. 2**O). The flattening and the calla lily cavosurface have made this tooth safer than in the traditional methods; however, it is not safe until the cusps are physically onlayed with restorative material.

CASE 3: THE UPPER FIRST MOLAR WITH A PORCELAIN-FUSED-TO-METAL CROWN

This case of the upper molar (**Fig. 3**A) highlights several issues encountered in real clinical cases. The tooth in this case has rotated and drifted mesially, has a PFM

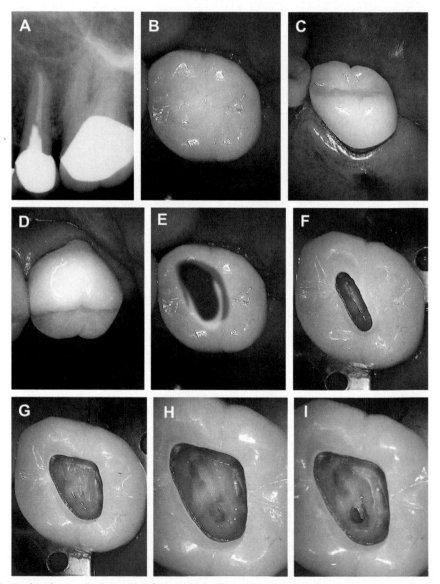

Fig. 3. (*A–P*) Case 3, the upper first molar with a PFM crown.

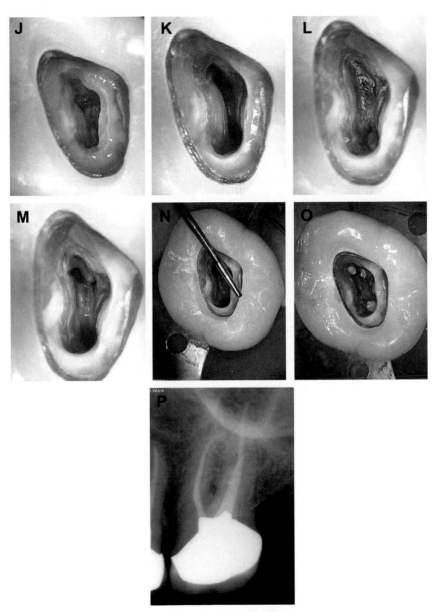

Fig. 3. (*continued*)

that obscures many of the normal anatomic landmarks, and has moderate calcification. The MB root has a cervical bend and a concurrent distal angle of entry to the MB system.

The preoperative occlusal view gives almost no indication of the underlying rotation or the multiplanar inclination of the underlying tooth (**Fig. 3**B). It is only through examination of the cervical outline that the clinician can gain some hints to the true orientation and inclination of the tooth and the modifications to the access that will be required. By observing the palatal view (**Fig. 3**C), the bulge of the palatal root can be prominently seen, and a hint as to the mesial inclination can be gained by observing the contour of the mesial contact reaching for the distal part of tooth No. 13. The preoperative buccal view (**Fig. 3**D) shows a reversal of the root prominences, with no evidence of the normally more prominent MB, yet a marked prominence of the DB, which is reflected both in the alveolar housing and the cervical contour of the PFM. This evidence suggests that the mesial of the tooth has rotated inward as it has drifted mesially. In the preoperative occlusal view, the translucency of the porcelain can often allow the clinician to look through to the opaque layer and better ascertain where at least the occlusal portion of the tooth mass is. The yellow outline form (**Fig. 3**E) shows a normal orientation on a maxillary first molar, with the mesial roughly paralleling the mesial of the crown, but authors are not accessing the crown; authors are accessing the root structure through the crown. The blue outline shows an appropriate rotation of the outline form along with a mesial and buccal translation in an attempt to compensate for the rotation and tipping of the underlying tooth structure. It is also increased in size to reflect the lower confidence in the true locations of the underlying tooth mass. The smaller black outline represents the expected outline form that is obtained once the clinician gains access to the underlying dentin map, and it is reflective of the more oval shape of the maxillary second molar pulp chamber. There is no green outline for this difficult type of case. The initial cut through porcelain and metal and slightly into dentin is oriented along the anticipated line connecting the MB and palatal (P) horns, generally the largest of the pulp horns (**Fig. 3**F). The access is liberally extended in the crown without progressing apically (**Fig. 3**G). A close-up shows a color change, whereby it would be reasonable to expect a P pulp horn (**Fig. 3**H). Careful apical progression through dentin exposes the chamber through the P horn, and the color map gives a visual cue as to the location of the MB horn as well (**Fig. 3**I). The tip of a CK bur is barely placed through the exposed P horn, dropping through the chamber roof, and is drawn around using the visual cues filtered through the expected chamber outline (black outline form mentioned earlier, **Fig. 3**J). **Fig. 3**K shows a considerable soffit over the P horn, less over the MB, and almost none over the DB. The buccal-most extent of the MB is carefully partially unroofed and troughed out to ensure that an additional MB canal is not present to the buccal, and a small amount of troughing and fluting slightly buccal of the palatal canal is done, because maxillary second molars occasionally harbors the MB2 canals in or near the P orifice (**Fig. 3**L). **Fig. 3**M shows the completed outline form ready for instrumentation. If the angle of entry to the DB is too constricted, a CK bur can be used to remove the small lip of dentin. The old residual DB horn can be seen when observed carefully. **Fig. 3**N shows the absolute sizes of the outline form through the PFM and the step in once the dentin is reached. **Fig. 3**O shows a slightly different view with a fairly dramatic step at the distal and palatal and a little-to-no step toward the MB. Thus, even with a fairly dramatic rotation and translation of the outline form, the access through the PFM was barely buccal and mesial enough. The final radiograph is shown in **Fig. 3**P.

CASE 4: MAXILLARY FIRST MOLAR WITH TYPICAL COMPLEXITY OF THE MB ROOT

A common criticism of these more-precise endodontic accesses is that they preclude PON location and discovery of deep anatomy. Yet there is no real evidence that generous outline forms actually facilitate discovery of coronal or deep anatomy. This can be confirmed by reviewing endodontic texts that continue to present clinical cases such as this fairly routine upper molar as anatomic oddities.

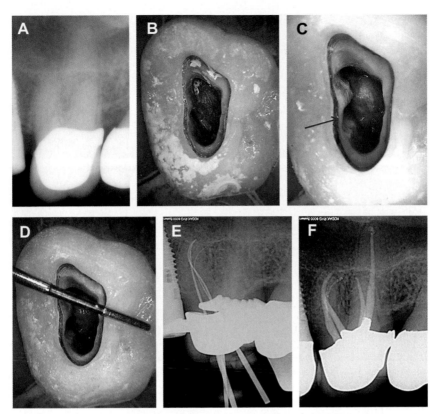

Fig. 4. (A–F) Maxillary first molar with a typical complexity of the MB root.

This case presents a stepped access on a somewhat calcific maxillary molar through a PFM (Fig. 4A). The initial outline form is on the larger side until the dentin is reached (Fig. 4B). Once the dentin is reached, the visual cues are followed as shown in case 6, slowly dissecting away just enough dentin to gain access. In this case, a cervical bulge shrouds the MB2 orifice, which is a fairly common finding in a maxillary molar. Instead of extending the entire mesial wall and unnecessarily removing irreplaceable PCD to gain access to the MB2 orifice, the mesial wall is slightly fluted as the MB2 is chased mesially before finally diving down the root (Fig. 4C). Fig. 4D shows the dimensions of the finished outline form using a 3-mm Marquis probe.

The canals are prepared, and a confluent MB/MB2 is noted. With this canal configuration, a deep split off the MB2 reaching the palatal is not an infrequent finding. This deep split is picked up by using a precurved file with a marked stopper, with the tip of the file directed along the palatal aspect of the MB2-prepared MB2 wall. Fig. 4E shows 3 instruments in the MB root: a No. 20 hand file in the MB orifice and 2 files (Nos. 20 and 10) in the MB2 orifice. The 2 No. 20 files can be seen to join, while the smaller No. 10 file curves off to a separate portal of exit. The final radiograph demonstrates the confluent prepared canals and the deep split likely filled with sealer (Fig. 4F).

Endodontic treatment is a balancing act. In the final analysis, the endodontic anatomy needs to be adequately addressed, requiring removal of dentin, which cannot possibly result in a stronger tooth. The authors believe that the endodontic

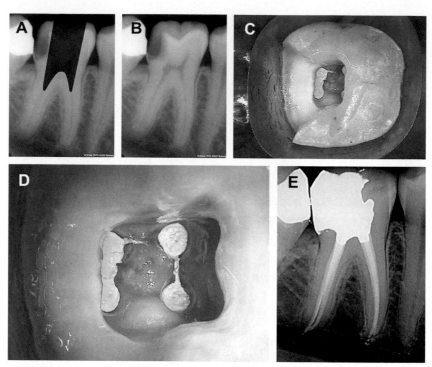

Fig. 5. (*A–E*) Caries-leveraged access in a lower first molar.

access has probed too far and that teeth are being needlessly weakened because of these larger outline forms, shapes, and the occult gouging that accompanies the traditional access technique and instrumentation. The clinician needs to be acutely aware of the biologic price of dentin removal and should always ask the question *"Do I really need to cut here?"*

CASE 5: CARIES-LEVERAGED ACCESS IN A LOWER FIRST MOLAR

Traditional endodontic access has paid little importance to the concept of directed dentin conservation, placing the operator's needs for facile access to the canal systems above the restoration needs and the tooth needs, when it is really a balance between these needs that is the objective. Traditionally, a case like this lower molar would have an endodontic access cut paying no importance to the decay on the distal, but instead, removing a substantial amount of the remaining healthy tooth structure (in the mesial region) to aid in accomplishing the endodontic objectives (**Fig. 5**A, B).

To avoid such a situation, the authors introduce the concept of caries- and filling-leveraged access, whereby existing restorative materials, decay, and less-strategic tooth structure are preferentially removed in favor of keeping tooth structure farther up on the hierarchy of tooth needs. Creativity and resourcefulness are the new directives. This concept leverages the availability of low- or zero-value tooth or restorative materials to skew the access and direct the conservation of dentin to where it is most important. In this case, there is distal decay, which is of zero value. The access is skewed distally, being almost entirely in the distal half of the tooth (**Fig. 5**C). A close-up of the chamber shows that the mesial wall, the mesial portion of the chamber

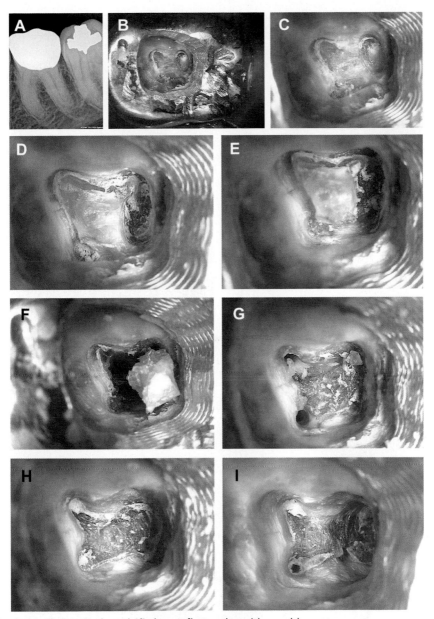

Fig. 6. (*A–O*) Case 6, the calcific lower first molar with a gold crown.

roof or soffit, as well as the mesial pulp horns are untouched and are left in their natural anatomic state (**Fig. 5**D). The undercut areas are cleaned out with prebent Maillefer micro-openers and Shepherd hook explorers. The final radiograph shows the completed case with an amalgam core that has been driven up into the mesial pulp horns (**Fig. 5**E). If traditional access had been cut in this tooth, the 3-dimensional ferrule in the most important walls, buccal and lingual, would have been insufficient to retain the tooth long term.

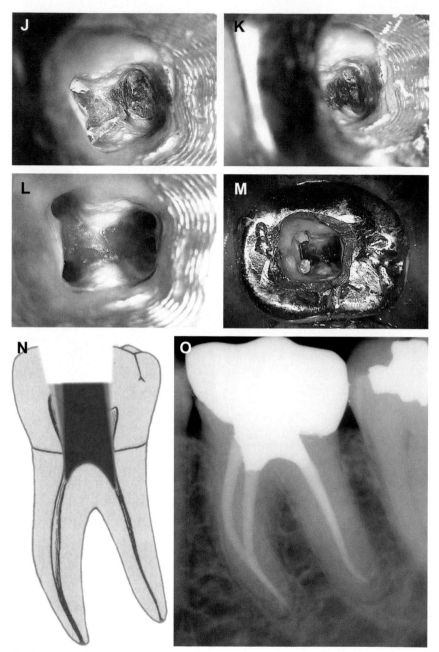

Fig. 6. (*continued*)

CASE 6: THE CALCIFIC LOWER FIRST MOLAR WITH A GOLD CROWN

The idea of using a round bur to drop in to a pulp chamber was put to test on a case such as a fairly routine lower molar (**Fig. 6**A). After a wide access was cut through the gold crown to the level at which dentin is encountered, the access was stepped in, and the color map was followed, leading to the first pulp tissue remnant (PTR) (**Fig. 6**B). The framework through which the color map and PTRs were interpreted was the outline of the pulp chamber when the patient was young (**Fig. 6**C). In this case, a pulp stone had been growing for decades and had obliterated the bulk of the lumen of the pulp chamber, leaving a periphery of PTRs that could be traced out with ultrasonics or CK burs.

Exploration is worthless with this case type because the bulk of the periphery sticks, leading to innumerable false positives, wasted time, and unnecessary digging that results in occult damage to the PCD. Instead, a moat is cut around the pulp stone. **Fig. 6**D shows the moat troughing around 3 of the 4 sides of this roughly trapezoidal chamber. The partial trough starts at the ML line angle and moves buccal to the MB line angle, turns about 90° distal toward the DB, turns another 90° at the DB line angle proceeding lingually, and terminates at the DL line angle. **Fig. 6**E shows the last leg of the moat connecting the DL to the ML.

A spoon excavator can usually pop the stone free (**Fig. 6**F). The chamber floor is inspected, revealing a small piece of necrotic pulp emanating from the MB and some residual stone stuck to the pulpal floor flowing down the distal system occluding access to that system (**Fig. 6**G). A mild amount of troughing reveals a fairly tenacious stone stuck partway down the distal system (**Fig. 6**H). Continued troughing begins to eliminate PTRs around several parts of the chamber periphery (**Fig. 6**I).

Troughing the distal system reveals a PTR surrounding the stone lodged in the distal system similar to the way in which the initial pulp stone occluded the pulp chamber (**Fig. 6**J). Again, the mental model is to identify the periphery of the stone by looking for color changes and PTRs that match the expected shape of lumen of the distal canal (**Fig. 6**K).

The cleaned-up and prepared chamber is shown in **Fig. 6**L. The obturated case was planned for a bonded amalgam repair of the access. As gold is not an etchable substrate, the cavosurface was left as a butt joint (**Fig. 6**M, N). The final radiograph is presented in **Fig. 6**O.

The strategy is to cut a larger-than-needed access through the dispensable restorative material only to the depth at which dentin is encountered. First cues in the color map should then be used to find the first PTRs, and slowly and carefully the dentin, pulp stones, and restoratives are dissected away to find the extent of the pulp chamber floor. By carefully tracing around the chamber floor, the PONs, which are almost invariably located at the periphery of the chamber floor, can be identified. Endodontic explorers are relics from the tactile-based world and have little value in the vision-based world in a case such as this.

FINAL NOTES: LOGISTICS OF THE CK APPROACH TO MOLAR ACCESS

1. You will notice that your measurement reference points may change; for example, in the past, the reference for the mesial canals was often the corresponding MB cusp. You may now find the reference more to the distal as you have preserved PCD and soffit dentin.
2. The simultaneous placement of 4 or 5 gutta-percha points for a cone fit radiograph in this more constricted access may require that some of the cones be cut back into the chamber to eliminate binding.
3. We recommend not removing the pulp tissue under the soffit until the obturation is finished; that way you only have to clean it up once.

Irrigation in Endodontics

Markus Haapasalo, DDS, PhD[a],*, Ya Shen, DDS, PhD[a],
Wei Qian, DDS, PhD[b], Yuan Gao, DDS, PhD[c]

KEYWORDS

• Endodontics • Irrigation • Root canal • Irrigant

The success of endodontic treatment depends on the eradication of microbes (if present) from the root-canal system and prevention of reinfection. The root canal is shaped with hand and rotary instruments under constant irrigation to remove the inflamed and necrotic tissue, microbes/biofilms, and other debris from the root-canal space. The main goal of instrumentation is to facilitate effective irrigation, disinfection, and filling. Several studies using advanced techniques such as microcomputed tomography (CT) scanning have demonstrated that proportionally large areas of the main root-canal wall remain untouched by the instruments,[1] emphasizing the importance of chemical means of cleaning and disinfecting all areas of the root canal (**Figs. 1** and **2**). There is no single irrigating solution that alone sufficiently covers all of the functions required from an irrigant. Optimal irrigation is based on the combined use of 2 or several irrigating solutions, in a specific sequence, to predictably obtain the goals of safe and effective irrigation. Irrigants have traditionally been delivered into the root-canal space using syringes and metal needles of different size and tip design. Clinical experience and research have shown, however, that this classic approach typically results in ineffective irrigation, particularly in peripheral areas such as anastomoses between canals, fins, and the most apical part of the main root canal. Therefore, many of the compounds used for irrigation have been chemically modified and several mechanical devices have been developed to improve the penetration and effectiveness of irrigation. This article summarizes the chemistry, biology, and procedures for safe and efficient irrigation and provides cutting-edge information on the most recent developments.

[a] Division of Endodontics, Department of Oral Biological & Medical Sciences, UBC Faculty of Dentistry, The University of British Columbia, 2199 Wesbrook Mall, Vancouver, BC, Canada V6T 1Z3
[b] Graduate Endodontics Program, Faculty of Dentistry, The University of British Columbia, 2199 Wesbrook Mall, Vancouver, BC, Canada V6T 1Z3
[c] State Key Laboratory of Oral Diseases, West China College & Hospital of Stomatology, Sichuan University, Chengdu, China
* Corresponding author.
E-mail address: markush@interchange.ubc.ca

Dent Clin N Am 54 (2010) 291–312
doi:10.1016/j.cden.2009.12.001
0011-8532/10/$ – see front matter © 2010 Elsevier Inc. All rights reserved.

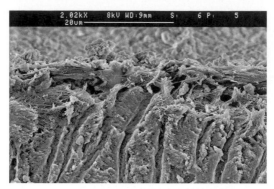

Fig. 1. A scanning electron microscopy image of dentin surface covered by predentin and other organic debris in an uninstrumented canal area.

GOALS OF IRRIGATION

Irrigation has a central role in endodontic treatment. During and after instrumentation, the irrigants facilitate removal of microorganisms, tissue remnants, and dentin chips from the root canal through a flushing mechanism (**Box 1**). Irrigants can also help prevent packing of the hard and soft tissue in the apical root canal and extrusion of infected material into the periapical area. Some irrigating solutions dissolve either organic or inorganic tissue in the root canal. In addition, several irrigating solutions have antimicrobial activity and actively kill bacteria and yeasts when introduced in direct contact with the microorganisms. However, several irrigating solutions also have cytotoxic potential, and they may cause severe pain if they gain access into the periapical tissues.[2] An optimal irrigant should have all or most of the positive characteristics listed in **Box 1**, but none of the negative or harmful properties. None of the available irrigating solutions can be regarded as optimal. Using a combination of products in the correct irrigation sequence contributes to a successful treatment outcome.

IRRIGATING SOLUTIONS
Sodium Hypochlorite

Sodium hypochlorite (NaOCl) is the most popular irrigating solution. NaOCl ionizes in water into Na^+ and the hypochlorite ion, OCl^-, establishing an equilibrium with

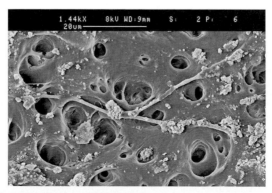

Fig. 2. Area of uninstrumented root-canal wall.

Box 1
Desired functions of irrigating solutions

- Washing action (helps remove debris)
- Reduce instrument friction during preparation (lubricant)
- Facilitate dentin removal (lubricant)
- Dissolve inorganic tissue (dentin)
- Penetrate to canal periphery
- Dissolve organic matter (dentin collagen, pulp tissue, biofilm)
- Kill bacteria and yeasts (also in biofilm)
- Do not irritate or damage vital periapical tissue, no caustic or cytotoxic effects
- Do not weaken tooth structure

---

hypochlorous acid (HOCl). At acidic and neutral pH, chlorine exists predominantly as HOCl, whereas at high pH of 9 and above, OCl⁻ predominates.[3] Hypochlorous acid is responsible for the antibacterial activity; the OCl⁻ ion is less effective than the undissolved HOCl. Hypochloric acid disrupts several vital functions of the microbial cell, resulting in cell death.[4,5]

NaOCl is commonly used in concentrations between 0.5% and 6%. It is a potent antimicrobial agent, killing most bacteria instantly on direct contact. It also effectively dissolves pulpal remnants and collagen, the main organic components of dentin. Hypochlorite is the only root-canal irrigant of those in general use that dissolves necrotic and vital organic tissue. It is difficult to imagine successful irrigation of the root canal without hypochlorite. Although hypochlorite alone does not remove the smear layer, it affects the organic part of the smear layer, making its complete removal possible by subsequent irrigation with EDTA or citric acid (CA). It is used as an unbuffered solution at pH 11 in the various concentrations mentioned earlier, or buffered with bicarbonate buffer (pH 9.0), usually as a 0.5% (Dakin solution) or 1% solution.[3] However, buffering does not seem to have any major effect on the properties of NaOCl, contrary to earlier belief.[6]

There is considerable variation in the literature regarding the antibacterial effect of NaOCl. In some articles hypochlorite is reported to kill the target microorganisms in seconds, even at low concentrations, although other reports have published considerably longer times for the killing of the same species.[7–10] Such differences are a result of confounding factors in some of the studies. The presence of organic matter during the killing experiments has a great effect on the antibacterial activity of NaOCl. Haapasalo and colleagues[11] showed that the presence of dentin caused marked delays in the killing of *Enterococcus faecalis* by 1% NaOCl. Many of the earlier studies were performed in the presence of an unknown amount of organic matter (eg, nutrient broth) or without controlling the pH of the culture, both of which affect the result. When the confounding factors are eliminated, it has been shown that NaOCl kills the target microorganisms rapidly even at low concentrations of less than 0.1%.[9,12] However, in vivo the presence of organic matter (inflammatory exudate, tissue remnants, microbial biomass) consumes NaOCl and weakens its effect. Therefore, continuous irrigation and time are important factors for the effectiveness of hypochlorite.

Byström and Sundqvist[13,14] studied the irrigation of root canals that were necrotic and contained a mixture of anaerobic bacteria. These investigators showed that using

0.5% or 5% NaOCl, with or without EDTA for irrigation, resulted in considerable reduction of bacterial counts in the canal when compared with irrigation with saline. However, it was difficult to render the canals completely free from bacteria, even after repeated sessions. Siqueira and colleagues[15] reported similar results using root canals infected with *E faecalis*. Both studies failed to show a significant difference in the antibacterial efficacy between the low and high concentrations of NaOCl. Contrary to these results, Clegg and colleagues,[16] in an ex vivo biofilm study, demonstrated a strong difference in the effectiveness against biofilm bacteria by 6% and 3% NaOCl, the higher concentration being more effective.

The weaknesses of NaOCl include the unpleasant taste, toxicity, and its inability to remove the smear layer (**Fig. 3**) by itself, as it dissolves only organic material.[17] The limited antimicrobial effectiveness of NaOCl in vivo is also disappointing. The poorer in vivo performance compared with in vitro is probably caused by problems in penetration to the most peripheral parts of the root-canal system such as fins, anastomoses, apical canal, lateral canals, and dentin canals. Also, the presence of inactivating substances such as exudate from the periapical area, pulp tissue, dentin collagen, and microbial biomass counteract the effectiveness of NaOCl.[11] Recently, it has been shown by in vitro studies that long-term exposure of dentin to a high concentration sodium hypochlorite can have a detrimental effect on dentin elasticity and flexural strength.[18,19] Although there are no clinical data on this phenomenon, it raises the question of whether hypochlorite in some situations may increase the risk of vertical root fracture.

In summary, sodium hypochlorite is the most important irrigating solution and the only one capable of dissolving organic tissue, including biofilm and the organic part of the smear layer. It should be used throughout the instrumentation phase. However, use of hypochlorite as the final rinse following EDTA or CA rapidly produces severe erosion of the canal-wall dentin and should probably be avoided.[20]

EDTA and CA

Complete cleaning of the root-canal system requires the use of irrigants that dissolve organic and inorganic material. As hypochlorite is active only against the former, other substances must be used to complete the removal of the smear layer and dentin debris. EDTA and CA effectively dissolve inorganic material, including hydroxyapatite.[21–24] They have little or no effect on organic tissue and alone they do not have antibacterial activity, despite some conflicting reports on EDTA. EDTA is most commonly

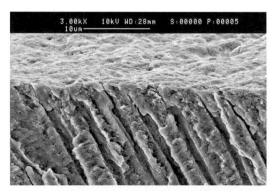

Fig. 3. Cross section of root dentin covered by the smear layer created by instrumentation. Notice smear plugs in dentin canals.

used as a 17% neutralized solution (disodium EDTA, pH 7), but a few reports have indicated that solutions with lower concentrations (eg, 10%, 5%, and even 1%) remove the smear layer equally well after NaOCl irrigation. Considering the high cost of EDTA, it may be worthwhile to consider using diluted EDTA. CA is also marketed and used in various concentrations, ranging from 1% to 50%, with a 10% solution being the most common. EDTA and CA are used for 2 to 3 minutes at the end of instrumentation and after NaOCl irrigation. Removal of the smear layer by EDTA or CA improves the antibacterial effect of locally used disinfecting agents in deeper layers of dentin.[25,26] EDTA and CA are manufactured as liquids and gels. Although there are no comparative studies about the effectiveness of liquid and gel products to demineralize dentin, it is possible that the small volume of the root canal (only a few microliters) contributes to a rapid saturation of the chemical and thereby loss of effectiveness. In such situations, the use of liquid products and continuous irrigation should be recommended.[27,28]

Chlorhexidine Digluconate

Chlorhexidine digluconate (CHX) is widely used in disinfection in dentistry because of its good antimicrobial activity.[29-31] It has gained considerable popularity in endodontics as an irrigating solution and as an intracanal medicament. CHX does not possess some of the undesired characteristics of sodium hypochlorite (ie, bad smell and strong irritation to periapical tissues). However, CHX has no tissue-dissolving capability and therefore it cannot replace sodium hypochlorite.

CHX permeates the microbial cell wall or outer membrane and attacks the bacterial cytoplasmic or inner membrane or the yeast plasma membrane. In high concentrations, CHX causes coagulation of intracellular components.[3] One of the reasons for the popularity of CHX is its substantivity (ie, continued antimicrobial effect), because CHX binds to hard tissue and remains antimicrobial. However, similar to other endodontic disinfecting agents, the activity of CHX depends on the pH and is also greatly reduced in the presence of organic matter.[31]

Several studies have compared the antibacterial effect of NaOCl and 2% CHX against intracanal infection and have shown little or no difference between their antimicrobial effectiveness.[32-35] Although bacteria may be killed by CHX, the biofilm and other organic debris are not removed by it. Residual organic tissue may have a negative effect on the quality of the seal by the permanent root filling, necessitating the use of NaOCl during instrumentation. However, CHX does not cause erosion of dentin like NaOCl does as the final rinse after EDTA, and therefore 2% CHX may be a good choice for maximized antibacterial effect at the end of the chemomechanical preparation.[36]

Most of the research on the use of CHX in endodontics is carried out using in vitro and ex vivo models and gram-positive test organisms, mostly *E faecalis*. It is therefore possible that the studies have given an overpositive picture of the usefulness of CHX as an antimicrobial agent in endodontics. More research is needed to identify the optimal irrigation regimen for various types of endodontic treatments. CHX is marketed as a water-based solution and as a gel (with Natrosol). Some studies have indicated that the CHX gel has a slightly better performance than the CHX liquid but the reasons for possible differences are not known.[37]

Other Irrigating Solutions

Other irrigating solutions used in endodontics have included sterile water, physiologic saline, hydrogen peroxide, urea peroxide, and iodine compounds. All of these except iodine compounds lack antibacterial activity when used alone, and they do not dissolve tissue either. Therefore there is no good reason for their use in canal irrigation in routine cases. In addition, water and saline solutions bear the risk of contamination if used from containers that have been opened more than once. Iodine potassium iodide (eg, 2% and 4%, respectively) has considerable antimicrobial activity but no tissue-dissolving capability[38,39] and it could be used at the end of the chemomechanical preparation like CHX. However, some patients are allergic to iodine, which must be taken into consideration.

Interactions Between Irrigating Solutions

Hypochlorite and EDTA are the 2 most commonly used irrigating solutions. As they have different characteristics and tasks, it has been tempting to use them as a mixture. However, EDTA (and CA) instantaneously reduces the amount of chlorine when mixed with sodium hypochlorite, resulting in the loss of NaOCl activity. Thus, these solutions should not be mixed.[40]

CHX has no tissue-dissolving activity and there have been efforts to combine CHX with hypochlorite for added benefits from the 2 solutions. However, CHX and NaOCl are not soluble in each other; a brownish-orange precipitate is formed when they are mixed (**Fig. 4**). The characteristics of the precipitate and the liquid phase have not been thoroughly examined, but the precipitate prevents the clinical use of the mixture. Atomic absorption spectrophotometry has indicated that the precipitate contains iron, which may be the reason for the orange development.[41] Presence of parachloroaniline, which may have mutagenic potential, has also been demonstrated in the precipitate.[42,43]

Mixing CHX and EDTA immediately produces a white precipitate (**Fig. 5**). Although the properties of the mixture and the cleared supernatant have not been thoroughly studied, it seems that the ability of EDTA to remove the smear layer is reduced.

Many clinicians mix NaOCl with hydrogen peroxide for root-canal irrigation. Despite more vigorous bubbling, the effectiveness of the mixture has not been shown to be

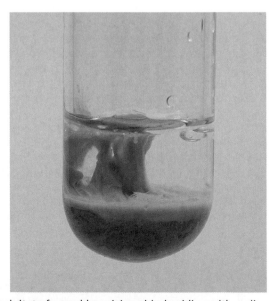

Fig. 4. Orange precipitate formed by mixing chlorhexidine with sodium hypochlorite.

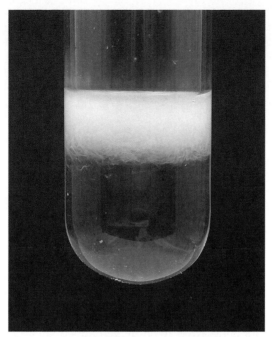

Fig. 5. Mixing sodium chlorhexidine with EDTA produces a white cloud and some precipitation.

better than that of NaOCl alone.[32] However, combining hydrogen peroxide with CHX in an ex vivo model[32,44] resulted in a considerable increase in the antibacterial activity of the mixture compared with the components alone in an infected dentin block. However, there are no data concerning the use or effectiveness of the mixture in clinical use.

Combination Products

Although some of the main irrigating solutions cannot be mixed without loss of activity or development of potentially toxic by-products, several combination products are on the market, many with some evidence of improved activity and function. Surface-active agents have been added to several different types of irrigants to lower their surface tension and to improve their penetration in the root canal. In the hope of better smear-layer removal, detergents have been added to some EDTA preparations (eg, SmearClear (**Fig. 6**))[45] and hypoclorite (eg, Chlor-XTRA (**Fig. 7**) and White King). Detergent addition has been shown to increase the speed of tissue dissolution by hypochlorite.[46] No data are available on whether dentin penetration is also improved. Recently, a few studies have been published in which the antibacterial activity of a chlorhexidine product with surface-active agents (CHX-Plus; see **Fig. 7**) has been compared with regular CHX, both with 2% chlorhexidine concentrations. The studies[47,48] have shown superior killing of planktonic and biofilm bacteria by the combination product. There are no studies about whether adding surface-active agents increases the risk of the irrigants escaping to the periapical area in clinical use.

MTAD (a mixture of tetracycline isomer, acid, and detergent, Biopure, Tulsa Dentsply, Tulsa, OK, USA) and Tetraclean are new combination products for root-canal irrigation that contain an antibiotic, doxycycline.[49–51] MTAD and Tetraclean are

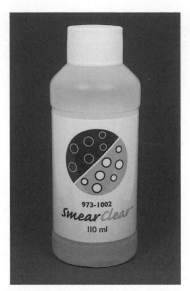

Fig. 6. SmearClear is a combination product containing EDTA and a detergent.

designed primarily for smear-layer removal with added antimicrobial activity. Both contain CA, doxycycline, and a detergent. They differ from each other in CA concentration and type of detergent included. They do not dissolve organic tissue and are intended for use at the end of chemomechanical preparation after sodium hypochlorite. Although earlier studies showed promising antibacterial effects by MTAD,[52,53] recent studies have indicated that an NaOCl/EDTA combination is equally or more effective

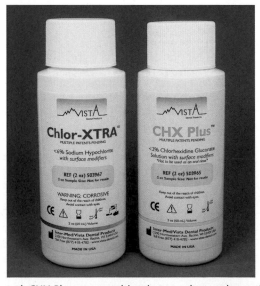

Fig. 7. Chlor-XTRA and CHX-Plus are combination products whose tissue dissolution or antibacterial properties have been improved by specific surface-active agents.

than NaOCl/MTAD.[54,55] Comparative studies on MATD and Tetraclean have indicated better antibacterial effects by the latter.[56] Although a mixture containing an antibiotic may have good short-term and long-term effects, concerns have been expressed regarding the use of tetracycline (doxycycline) because of possible resistance to the antibiotic and staining of the tooth hard tissue, which has been demonstrated by exposure to light in an in vitro expreriment.[57] However, no report of in vivo staining has been published.

CHALLENGES OF IRRIGATION
Smear Layer

Removal of the smear layer is straightforward and predictable when the correct irrigants are used. Relying on EDTA alone or other irrigants with activity against the inorganic matter only, however, results in incomplete removal of the layer. Therefore, use of hypochlorite during instrumentation cannot be omitted (**Fig. 8**). The smear layer is created only on areas touched by the instruments. Delivery of irrigants to these areas is usually unproblematic, with the possible exception of the most apical canal, depending on canal morphology and the techniques/equipment used for irrigation. However, careless irrigation, with needles introduced only to the coronal and middle parts of the root canal, is likely to result in incomplete removal of the smear layer in the apical root canal.

Dentin Erosion

One of the goals of endodontic treatment is to protect the tooth structure so that the physical procedures and chemical treatments do not cause weakening of the dentin/root. Erosion of dentin has not been studied much; however, there is a general consensus that dentin erosion may be harmful and should be avoided. A few studies have shown that long-term exposure to high concentrations of hypochlorite can lead to considerable reduction in the flexural strength and elastic modus of dentin.[19] These studies have been performed in vitro using dentin blocks, which may allow artificially deep penetration of hypoclorite into dentin. However, even short-term irrigation with hypochlorite after EDTA or CA at the end of chemomechanical preparation causes strong erosion of the canal-wall surface dentin (**Fig. 9**).[20] Although it is not known for sure whether surface erosion is a negative issue or if, for example, it could improve dentin bonding for posts, it is the authors' opinion that hypochlorite irrigation after

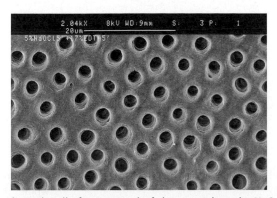

Fig. 8. Instrumented canal wall after removal of the smear layer by NaOCl and EDTA.

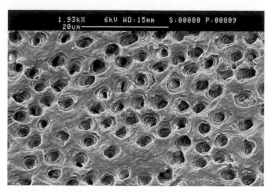

Fig. 9. Considerable erosion of canal-wall dentin occurs when hypochlorite is used after EDTA or CA.

demineralization agents should be avoided. Instead, chlorhexidine irrigation could be used for additional disinfection at the end of the treatment.

Cleaning of Uninstrumented Parts of the Root-canal System

Irrigation is most feasible in the instrumented areas because the irrigation needle can follow the smooth path created by the instruments. Cleaning and removing of necrotic tissue, debris, and biofilms from untouched areas rely completely on chemical means, and sufficient use of sodium hypochlorite is the key factor in obtaining the desired results in these areas (**Fig. 10**). A recent study showed that untouched areas, in particular anastomoses between canals, are frequently packed with debris during instrumentation.[58] Visibility in micro-CT scans indicates that the debris also contain a considerable proportion of inorganic material (**Fig. 11**). Although at present it is not known how these debris can best be removed (if at all), it is likely that physical agitation (eg, ultrasound) and the use of demineralizing agents are needed in addition to hypochlorite.

Biofilm

Biofilm (**Fig. 12**) can be removed or eliminated through the following methods: mechanical removal by instruments (effective only in some areas of the root canal);

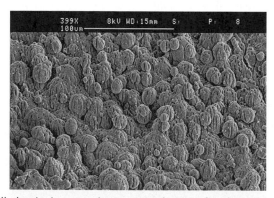

Fig. 10. Canal-wall dentin in an uninstrumented area after hypochlorite irrigation has removed (dissolved) tissue remnants and predentin, revealing the large calcospherites that have already joined mineralized dentin.

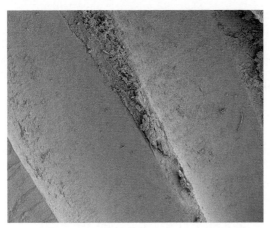

Fig. 11. An anastomosis between 2 joining canals has been packed with debris during rotary instrumentation.

dissolution by hypochlorite; and detachment by ultrasonic energy. Other chemical means, such as chlorhexidine, can kill biofilm bacteria if allowed a long enough contact time. However, as they lack tissue-dissolving ability, the dead microbial biomass stays in the canal if not removed mechanically or dissolved by hypochlorite. Any remaining organic matter, microbes, or vital or necrotic tissue jeopardizes the integrity of the seal of the root filling. Therefore the goal of the treatment is not only to kill the microbes in the root canal but also to remove them as completely as possible.

Safety versus Effectiveness in the Apical Root Canal

Irrigation must maintain a balance between 2 important goals: safety and effectiveness. This point is particularly true with the most important irrigant, sodium hypochlorite, but other irrigants can also cause pain and other problems if they gain access to the periapical tissues. Effectiveness is often jeopardized in the apical root canal by restricting anatomy and valid safety concerns. However, the eradication of the microbes in the apical canal should be of key importance to the success of endodontic

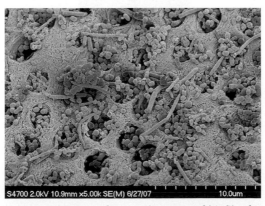

Fig. 12. Bacteria growing on dentin surface; early stages of biofilm formation.

treatment. Sufficient exchange of hypochlorite and other irrigants in this area while keeping the apical pressure of the solutions minimal is the obvious goal of irrigation of the apical root canal. A better understanding of fluid dynamics and the development of new needle designs and equipment for irrigant delivery are the 2 important areas to deal with in the challenges of irrigating the most apical part of the canal. These areas are discussed in the following sections.

COMPUTATIONAL FLUID DYNAMICS IN THE ROOT-CANAL SPACE

Computational fluid dynamics (CFD) is a new approach in endodontic research to improve our understanding of fluid dynamics in the special anatomic environment of the root canal. Fluid flow is commonly studied in 1 of 3 ways: experimental fluid dynamics; theoretic fluid dynamics; and computational fluid dynamics (**Fig. 13**). CFD is the science that focuses on predicting fluid flow and related phenomena by solving the mathematical equations that govern these processes. Numerical and experimental approaches play complementary roles in the investigation of fluid flow. Experimental studies have the advantage of physical realism; once the numerical model is experimentally validated, it can be used to theoretically simulate various conditions and perform parametric investigations. CFD can be used to evaluate and predict specific parameters, such as the streamline (**Fig. 14**), velocity distribution of irrigant flow in the root canal (**Fig. 15**), wall flow pressure, and wall shear stress on the root-canal wall, which are difficult to measure in vivo because of the microscopic size of the root canals.

In CFD studies, no single turbulence model is universally accepted for different types of flow environments. The use of an unsuitable turbulence model may lead to potential numerical errors and affect CFD results.[59] Gao and colleagues[60] found that CFD analysis based on a shear stress transport (SST) κ-ω turbulence model

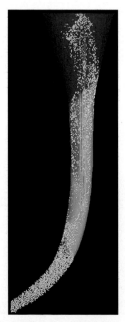

Fig. 13. Particle tracking during irrigation simulated by a CFD model.

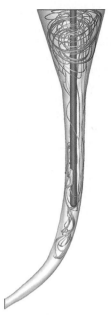

Fig. 14. Streamline provides visualization of the irrigant flow in the canal.

was in close agreement with the in vitro irrigation model. CFD based on an SST κ-ω turbulence model has the potential to serve as a platform for the study of root-canal irrigation.

The irrigant velocity on the canal wall is considered a highly significant factor in determining the replacement of the irrigant in certain parts of the root canal and

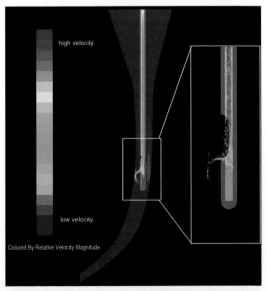

Fig. 15. Velocity contour and vectors colored by velocity magnitude in an SST κ-ω turbulence model. High-velocity flow seen in the needle lumen and in the area of the side vent.

in the flush effect, therefore directly influencing the effectiveness of irrigation.[61] In a turbulent flow, there is a viscous sublayer that is a thin region next to a wall, typically only 1% of the boundary-layer thickness, in which turbulent mixing is impeded and transport occurs partly or, as the limit of the wall is approached, entirely by viscous diffusion.[62] From turbulent structure measurements of pipe flow, the regions of maximum production and maximum dissipation are just outside the viscous sub-layer.[63] Hence, the fastest flow is found in the turbulent boundary, whereas the minimum velocity is observed on the wall of all root-canal irrigations. Some of the goals of CFD studies in endodontics are to improve needle-tip design for effective and safe delivery of the irrigant and to optimize the exchange of irrigating solutions in the peripheral parts of the canal system.

IRRIGATION DEVICES AND TECHNIQUES

The effectiveness and safety of irrigation depends on the means of delivery. Tradition-ally, irrigation has been performed with a plastic syringe and an open-ended needle into the canal space. An increasing number of novel needle-tip designs and equipment are emerging in an effort to better address the challenges of irrigation.

Syringes

Plastic syringes of different sizes (1–20 mL) are most commonly used for irrigation (**Fig. 16**). Although large-volume syringes potentially allow some time-savings, they are more difficult to control for pressure and accidents may happen. Therefore, to maximize safety and control, use of 1- to 5-mL syringes is recommended instead of the larger ones. All syringes for endodontic irrigation must have a Luer-Lok design. Because of the chemical reactions between many irrigants, separate syringes should be used for each solution.

Needles

Although 25-gauge needles were commonplace for endodontic irrigation a few years ago, they were first replaced by 27-G needles, now 30-G and even 31-G needles are taking over for routine use in irrigation. As 27 G corresponds to International Standards

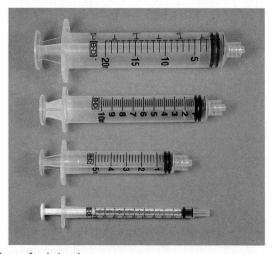

Fig. 16. Plastic syringes for irrigation.

Organization size 0.42 and 30 G to size 0.31, smaller needle sizes are preferred. Several studies have shown that the irrigant has only a limited effect beyond the tip of the needle because of the dead-water zone or sometimes air bubbles in the apical root canal, which prevent apical penetration of the solution. However, although the smaller needles allow delivery of the irrigant close to the apex, this is not without safety concerns. Several modifications of the needle-tip design have been introduced in recent years to facilitate effectiveness and minimize safety risks (**Figs. 17** and **18**). There are few comparative data about the effect of needle design on irrigation effectiveness; it is hoped that ongoing CFD and clinical studies will change this situation.

Gutta-percha Points

The recognition of the difficulty of apical canal irrigation has led to various innovative techniques to facilitate the penetration of solutions in the canal. One of these includes the use of apically fitting gutta-percha cones in an up-and-down motion at the working length. Although this facilitates the exchange of the apical solution, the overall volume of fresh solution in the apical canal is likely to remain small. However, the benefits of gutta-percha point assisted irrigation have been shown in 2 recent studies.[64,65]

EndoActivator

EndoActivator (Advanced Endodontics, Santa Barbara, CA, USA) is a new type of irrigation facilitator. It is based on sonic vibration (up to 10,000 cpm) of a plastic tip in the root canal. The system has 3 different sizes of tips that are easily attached (snap-on) to the handpiece that creates the sonic vibrations (**Fig. 19**). EndoActivator does not deliver new irrigant to the canal but it facilitates the penetration and renewal of the irrigant in the canal. Two recent studies have indicated that the use of EndoActivator facilitates irrigant penetration and mechanical cleansing compared with needle irrigation, with no increase in the risk of irrigant extrusion through the apex.[66,67]

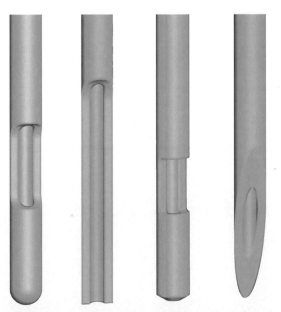

Fig. 17. Four different needle designs, produced by computerized mesh models based on true and virtual needles.

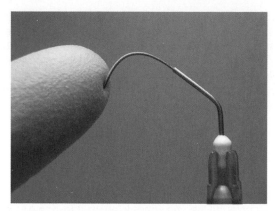

Fig. 18. Flexiglide needle for irrigation also easily follows curved canals.

Vibringe

Vibringe (Vibringe BV, Amsterdam, The Netherlands) is a new sonic irrigation system that combines battery-driven vibrations (9000 cpm) with manually operated irrigation of the root canal (**Fig. 20**). Vibringe uses the traditional type of syringe/needle delivery but adds sonic vibration. No studies can be found on Medline.

RinsEndo

The RinsEndo system (Durr Dental Co) is based on a pressure-suction mechanism with approximately 100 cycles per minute.[68] A study of the safety of several irrigation systems reported that the risk of overirrigation was comparable with manual and RinsEndo irrigation, but higher than with EndoActivator or the EndoVac system.[67] Not enough data are available to draw conclusions about the benefits and possible risks of the RinsEndo system.

EndoVac

EndoVac (Discus Dental, Culver City, CA, USA) represents a novel approach to irrigation as, instead of delivering the irrigant through the needle, the EndoVac system is based on a negative-pressure approach whereby the irrigant placed in the pulp chamber is sucked down the root canal and back up again through a thin needle with a special design (**Fig. 21**). There is evidence that, compared with traditional needle irrigation and some other systems, the EndoVac system lowers the risks associated with irrigation close to the apical foramen considerably.[67] Another advantage of the reversed flow of irrigants may be good apical cleaning at the 1-mm level and a strong antibacterial effect when hypochlorite is used, as shown by recent studies.[69,70]

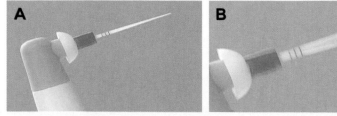

Fig. 19. (*A*) EndoActivator with the large (*blue*) plastic tip. (*B*) Same tip in sonic motion.

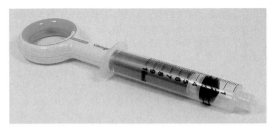

Fig. 20. Vibringe irrigator creates sonic vibrations in the syringe and needle.

Ultrasound

The use of ultrasonic energy for cleaning of the root canal and to facilitate disinfection has a long history in endodontics. The comparative effectiveness of ultrasonics and hand-instrumentation techniques has been evaluated in several earlier studies.[71–74] Most of these studies concluded that ultrasonics, together with an irrigant, contributed to a better cleaning of the root-canal system than irrigation and hand-instrumentation alone. Cavitation and acoustic streaming of the irrigant contribute to the biologic-chemical activity for maximum effectiveness.[75] Analysis of the physical mechanisms of the hydrodynamic response of an oscillating ultrasonic file suggested that stable and transient cavitation of a file, steady streaming, and cavitation microstreaming all contribute to the cleaning of the root canal.[76] Ultrasonic files must have free movement in the canal without making contact with the canal wall to work effectively.[77] Several studies have indicated the importance of ultrasonic preparation for optimal

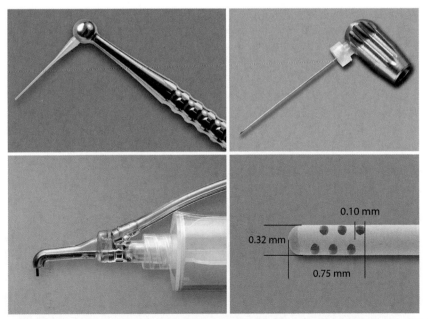

Fig. 21. EndoVac system uses negative pressure to make safe and effective irrigation of the most apical canal possible. The irrigant in the pulp chamber is sucked down the root canal and back up again via the needle, opposite to the classic method of irrigation.

debridement of anastomoses between double canals, isthmuses, and fins.[78–80] The effectiveness of ultrasonics in the elimination of bacteria and dentin debris from the canals has been shown by several studies.[81–85] However, not all studies have supported these findings.[80]

Van der Sluis and colleagues[84] suggested that a smooth wire during ultrasonic irrigation is as effective as a size 15 K-file in the removal of artificially placed dentin debris in grooves in simulated root canals in resin blocks. It is possible that preparation complications are less likely to occur with an ultrasonic tip with a smooth, inactive surface.

SUMMARY

Irrigation has a key role in successful endodontic treatment. Although hypochlorite is the most important irrigating solution, no single irrigant can accomplish all the tasks required by irrigation. Detailed understanding of the mode of action of various solutions is important for optimal irrigation. New developments such as CFD and mechanical devices will help to advance safe and effective irrigation.

ACKNOWLEDGMENTS

The authors would like to thank Ingrid Ellis for her editorial assistance in the final preparation of this manuscript.

REFERENCES

1. Peters OA, Schönenberger K, Laib A. Effects of four Ni-Ti preparation techniques on root canal geometry assessed by micro computed tomography. Int Endod J 2001;34:221–30.
2. Hülsmann M, Hahn W. Complications during root canal irrigation: literature review and case reports [review]. Int Endod J 2000;33:186–93.
3. Mcdonnell G, Russell D. Antiseptics and disinfectants: activity, action, and resistance. Clin Microbiol Rev 1999;12:147–79.
4. Barrette WC Jr, Hannum DM, Wheeler WD, et al. General mechanism for the bacterial toxicity of hypochlorous acid: abolition of ATP production. Biochemistry 1989;28:9172–8.
5. McKenna SM, Davies KJA. The inhibition of bacterial growth by hypochlorous acid. Biochem J 1988;254:685–92.
6. Zehnder M, Kosicki D, Luder H, et al. Tissue-dissolving capacity and antibacterial effect of buffered and unbuffered hypochlorite solutions. Oral Surg Oral Med Oral Pathol Oral Radiol Endod 2002;94:756–62.
7. Gomes BP, Ferraz CC, Vianna ME, et al. In vitro antimicrobial activity of several concentrations of sodium hypochlorite and chlorhexidine gluconate in the elimination of Enterococcus faecalis. Int Endod J 2001;34:424–8.
8. Radcliffe CE, Potouridou L, Qureshi R, et al. Antimicrobial activity of varying concentrations of sodium hypochlorite on the endodontic microorganisms Actinomyces israelii, A. naeslundii, Candida albicans and Enterococcus faecalis. Int Endod J 2004;37:438–46.
9. Vianna ME, Gomes BP, Berber VB, et al. In vitro evaluation of the antimicrobial activity of chlorhexidine and sodium hypochlorite. Oral Surg Oral Med Oral Pathol Oral Radiol Endod 2004;97:79–84.
10. Waltimo TM, Ørstavik D, Siren EK, et al. In vitro susceptibility of Candida albicans to four disinfectants and their combinations. Int Endod J 1999;32:421–9.

11. Haapasalo HK, Siren EK, Waltimo TM, et al. Inactivation of local root canal medicaments by dentine: an in vitro study. Int Endod J 2000;33:126–31.
12. Portenier I, Waltimo T, Ørstavik D, et al. The susceptibility of starved, stationary phase, and growing cells of Enterococcus faecalis to endodontic medicaments. J Endod 2005;31:380–6.
13. Byström A, Sundqvist G. Bacteriologic evaluation of the effect of 0.5 percent sodium hypochlorite in endodontic therapy. Oral Surg Oral Med Oral Pathol 1983;55:307–12.
14. Byström A, Sundqvist G. The antibacterial action of sodium hypochlorite and EDTA in 60 cases of endodontic therapy. Int Endod J 1985;18:35–40.
15. Siqueira JF Jr, Rocas IN, Santos SR, et al. Efficacy of instrumentation techniques and irrigation regimens in reducing the bacterial population within root canals. J Endod 2002;28:181–4.
16. Clegg MS, Vertucci FJ, Walker C, et al. The effect of exposure to irrigant solutions on apical dentin biofilms in vitro. J Endod 2006;32:434–7.
17. Spångberg L, Engström B, Langeland K. Biologic effects of dental materials. 3. Toxicity and antimicrobial effect of endodontic antiseptics in vitro. Oral Surg Oral Med Oral Pathol 1973;36:856–71.
18. Sim TP, Knowles JC, Ng YL, et al. Effect of sodium hypochlorite on mechanical properties of dentine and tooth surface strain. Int Endod J 2001;34:120–32.
19. Marending M, Luder HU, Brunner TJ, et al. Effect of sodium hypochlorite on human root dentine–mechanical, chemical and structural evaluation. Int Endod J 2007;40:786–93.
20. Niu W, Yoshioka T, Kobayashi C, et al. A scanning electron microscopic study of dentinal erosion by final irrigation with EDTA and NaOCl solutions. Int Endod J 2002;35:934–9.
21. Czonstkowsky M, Wilson EG, Holstein FA. The smear layer in endodontics. Dent Clin North Am 1990;34:13–25.
22. Baumgartner JC, Brown CM, Mader CL, et al. A scanning electron microscopic evaluation of root canal debridement using saline, sodium hypochlorite, and citric acid. J Endod 1984;10:525–31.
23. Baumgartner JC, Mader CL. A scanning electron microscopic evaluation of four root canal irrigation regimens. J Endod 1987;13:147–57.
24. Loel DA. Use of acid cleanser in endodontic therapy. J Am Dent Assoc 1975;90: 148–51.
25. Haapasalo M, Ørstavik D. In vitro infection and disinfection of dentinal tubules. J Dent Res 1987;66:1375–9.
26. Ørstavik D, Haapasalo M. Disinfection by endodontic irrigants and dressings of experimentally infected dentinal tubules. Endod Dent Traumatol 1990;6:142–9.
27. Hülsmann M, Heckendorff M, Lennon A. Chelating agents in root canal treatment: mode of action and indications for their use. Int Endod J 2003;36:810–30.
28. Zehnder M. Root canal irrigants. J Endod 2006;32:389–98.
29. Russell AD. Activity of biocides against mycobacteria. Soc Appl Bacteriol Symp Ser 1996;25:87S–101S.
30. Shaker LA, Dancer BN, Russell AD, et al. Emergence and development of chlorhexidine resistance during sporulation of Bacillus subtilis 168. FEMS Microbiol Lett 1988;51:73–6.
31. Russell AD, Day MJ. Antibacterial activity of chlorhexidine. J Hosp Infect 1993;25: 229–38.
32. Heling I, Chandler NP. Antimicrobial effect of irrigant combinations within dentinal tubules. Int Endod J 1998;31:8–14.

33. Vahdaty A, Pitt Ford TR, Wilson RF. Efficacy of chlorhexidine in disinfecting dentinal tubules in vitro. Endod Dent Traumatol 1993;9:243–8.
34. Buck RA, Eleazer PD, Staat RH, et al. Effectiveness of three endodontic irrigants at various tubular depths in human dentin. J Endod 2001;27:206–8.
35. Jeansonne MJ, White RR. A comparison of 2.0% chlorhexidine gluconate and 5.25% sodium hypochlorite as antimicrobial endodontic irrigants. J Endod 1994;20:276–8.
36. Zamany A, Safavi K, Spångberg LS. The effect of chlorhexidine as an endodontic disinfectant. Oral Surg Oral Med Oral Pathol Oral Radiol Endod 2003;96:578–81.
37. Ferraz CC, Gomes BP, Zaia AA, et al. In vitro assessment of the antimicrobial action and the mechanical ability of chlorhexidine gel as an endodontic irrigant. J Endod 2001;27:452–5.
38. Gottardi W. Iodine and iodine compounds. In: Block SS, editor. Disinfection, sterilization, and preservation. 4th edition. Philadelphia: Lea & Febiger; 1991. p. 152–66.
39. Molander A, Reit C, Dahlen G. The antimicrobial effect of calcium hydroxide in root canals pretreated with 5% iodine potassium iodide. Endod Dent Traumatol 1999;15:205–9.
40. Zehnder M, Schmidlin P, Sener B, et al. Chelation in root canal therapy reconsidered. J Endod 2005;31:817–20.
41. Marchesan MA, Pasternak Junior B, Afonso MM, et al. Chemical analysis of the flocculate formed by the association of sodium hypochlorite and chlorhexidine. Oral Surg Oral Med Oral Pathol Oral Radiol Endod 2007;103:103–5.
42. Basrani BR, Manek S, Sodhi RN, et al. Interaction between sodium hypochlorite and chlorhexidine gluconate. J Endod 2007;33:966–9.
43. Basrani BR, Manek S, Fillery E. Using diazotization to characterize the effect of heat or sodium hypochlorite on 2.0% chlorhexidine. J Endod 2009;35:1296–9.
44. Steinberg D, Heling I, Daniel I, et al. Antibacterial synergistic effect of chlorhexidine and hydrogen peroxide against *Streptococcus sobrinus, Streptococcus faecalis* and *Staphylococcus aureus*. J Oral Rehabil 1999;26:151–6.
45. Dunavant TR, Regan JD, Glickman GN, et al. Comparative evaluation of endodontic irrigants against *Enterococcus faecalis* biofilms. J Endod 2006;32:527–31.
46. Clarkson RM, Moule AJ, Podlich H, et al. Dissolution of porcine incisor pulps in sodium hypochlorite solutions of varying compositions and concentrations. Aust Dent J 2006;51:245–51.
47. Shen Y, Qian W, Chung C, et al. Evaluation of the effect of two chlorhexidine preparations on biofilm bacteria in vitro: a three-dimensional quantitative analysis. J Endod 2009;35:981–5.
48. Williamson AE, Cardon JW, Drake DR. Antimicrobial susceptibility of monoculture biofilms of a clinical isolate of *Enterococcus faecalis*. J Endod 2009;35:95–7.
49. Torabinejad M, Khademi AA, Babagoli J, et al. A new solution for the removal of the smear layer. J Endod 2003;29:170–5.
50. Torabinejad M, Cho Y, Khademi AA, et al. The effect of various concentrations of sodium hypochlorite on the ability of MTAD to remove the smear layer. J Endod 2003;29:233–9.
51. Giardino L, Ambu E, Becce C, et al. Surface tension comparison of four common root canal irrigants and two new irrigants containing antibiotic. J Endod 2006;32:1091–3.
52. Shabahang S, Pouresmail M, Torabinejad M. In vitro antimicrobial efficacy of MTAD and sodium. J Endod 2003;29:450–2.

53. Shabahang S, Torabinejad M. Effect of MTAD on *Enterococcus faecalis*-contaminated root canals of extracted human teeth. J Endod 2003;29:576–9.
54. Kho P, Baumgartner JC. A comparison of the antimicrobial efficacy of NaOCl/Biopure MTAD versus NaOCl/EDTA against *Enterococcus faecalis*. J Endod 2006; 32:652–5.
55. Baumgartner JC, Johal S, Marshall JG. Comparison of the antimicrobial efficacy of 1.3% NaOCl/BioPure MTAD to 5.25% NaOCl/15% EDTA for root canal irrigation. J Endod 2007;33:48–51.
56. Giardino L, Ambu E, Savoldi E, et al. Comparative evaluation of antimicrobial efficacy of sodium hypochlorite, MTAD, and Tetraclean against *Enterococcus faecalis* biofilm. J Endod 2007;33:852–5.
57. Tay FR, Mazzoni A, Pashley DH, et al. Potential iatrogenic tetracycline staining of endodontically treated teeth via NaOCl/MTAD irrigation: a preliminary report. J Endod 2006;32:354–8.
58. Paqué F, Laib A, Gautschi H, et al. Hard-tissue debris accumulation analysis by high-resolution computed tomography scans. J Endod 2009;35:1044–7.
59. van Ertbruggen C, Corieri P, Theunissen R, et al. Validation of CFD predictions of flow in a 3D alveolated bend with experimental data. J Biomech 2008;41: 399–405.
60. Gao Y, Haapasalo M, Shen Y, et al. Development and validation of a three-dimensional computational fluid dynamics model of root canal irrigation. J Endod 2009; 35:1282–7.
61. Boutsioukis C, Lambrianidis T, Kastrinakis E, et al. Measurement of pressure and flow rates during irrigation of a root canal ex vivo with three endodontic needles. Int Endod J 2007;40:504–13.
62. Townsend AA. The structure of turbulent shear flow. Cambridge: Cambridge University Press; 1976. p. 429.
63. Du Y, Karniadakis GE. Suppressing wall turbulence by means of a transverse traveling wave. Science 2000;288:1230–4.
64. McGill S, Gulabivala K, Mordan N, et al. The efficacy of dynamic irrigation using a commercially available system (RinsEndo) determined by removal of a collagen 'bio-molecular film' from an ex vivo model. Int Endod J 2008;41:602–8.
65. Huang TY, Gulabivala K, Ng Y- L. A bio-molecular film ex-vivo model to evaluate the influence of canal dimensions and irrigation variables on the efficacy of irrigation. Int Endod J 2008;41:60–71.
66. Townsend C, Maki J. An in vitro comparison of new irrigation and agitation techniques to ultrasonic agitation in removing bacteria from a simulated root canal. J Endod 2009;35:1040–3.
67. Desai P, Himel V. Comparative safety of various intracanal irrigation systems. J Endod 2009;35:545–9.
68. Hauser V, Braun A, Frentzen M. Penetration depth of a dye marker into dentine using a novel hydrodynamic system (RinsEndo). Int Endod J 2007;40:644–52.
69. Hockett JL, Dommisch JK, Johnson JD, et al. Antimicrobial efficacy of two irrigation techniques in tapered and nontapered canal preparations: an in vitro study. J Endod 2008;34:1374–7.
70. Nielsen BA, Craig Baumgartner J. Comparison of the EndoVac system to needle irrigation of root canals. J Endod 2007;33:611–5.
71. Plotino G, Pameijer CH, Grande NM, et al. Ultrasonics in endodontics: a review of the literature. J Endod 2007;33:81–95.
72. Martin H. Ultrasonic disinfection of the root canal. Oral Surg Oral Med Oral Pathol 1976;42:92–9.

73. Cunningham W, Martin H, Forrest W. Evaluation of root canal debridement by the endosonic ultrasonic synergistic system. Oral Surg Oral Med Oral Pathol 1982; 53:401–4.
74. Cunningham W, Martin H, Pelleu G, et al. A comparison of antimicrobial effectiveness of endosonic and hand root canal therapy. Oral Surg Oral Med Oral Pathol 1982;54:238–41.
75. Martin H, Cunningham W. Endosonics–the ultrasonic synergistic system of endodontics. Endod Dent Traumatol 1985;1:201–6.
76. Roy RA, Ahmad M, Crum LA. Physical mechanisms governing the hydrodynamic response of an oscillating ultrasonic file. Int Endod J 1994;27:197–207.
77. Lumley PJ, Walmsley AD, Walton RE, et al. Effect of pre-curving endosonic files on the amount of debris and smear layer remaining in curved root canals. J Endod 1992;18:616–9.
78. Goodman A, Reader A, Beck M, et al. An in vitro comparison of the efficacy of the step-back technique versus a step-back ultrasonic technique in human mandibular molars. J Endod 1985;11:249–56.
79. Archer R, Reader A, Nist R, et al. An in vivo evaluation of the efficacy of ultrasound after stepback preparation in mandibular molars. J Endod 1992;18: 549–52.
80. Sjögren U, Sundqvist G. Bacteriologic evaluation of ultrasonic root canal instrumentation. Oral Surg Oral Med Oral Pathol 1987;63:366–70.
81. Spoleti P, Siragusa M, Spoleti MJ. Bacteriological evaluation of passive ultrasonic activation. J Endod 2002;29:12–4.
82. Sabins RA, Johnson JD, Hellstein JW. A comparison of the cleaning efficacy of short term sonic and ultrasonic passive irrigation after hand instrumentation in molar root canals. J Endod 2003;29:674–8.
83. Lee SJ, Wu MK, Wesselink PR. The effectiveness of syringe irrigation and ultrasonics to remove debris from simulated irregularities within prepared root canal walls. Int Endod J 2004;37:672–8.
84. Van der Sluis LW, Wu MK, Wesselink PR. A comparison between a smooth wire and a K-file in removing artificially placed dentine debris from root canals in resin blocks during ultrasonic irrigation. Int Endod J 2005;38:593–6.
85. Van der Sluis LW, Wu MK, Wesselink PR. The evaluation of removal of calcium hydroxide paste from an artificial standardized groove in the apical root canal using different irrigation methodologies. Int Endod J 2007;40:52–7.

Treatment of the Immature Tooth with a Non–Vital Pulp and Apical Periodontitis

Martin Trope, DMD[a,b,*]

KEYWORDS

- Sodium hypochlorite • Calcium hydroxide
- Revascularization • Periodontitis • Mineral trioxide aggregate

The immature root with a necrotic pulp and apical periodontitis (**Fig. 1**) presents multiple challenges to successful treatment.

1. The infected root canal space cannot be disinfected with the standard root canal protocol with the aggressive use of endodontic files.
2. Once the microbial phase of the treatment is complete, filling the root canal is difficult because the open apex provides no barrier for stopping the root filling material before impinging on the periodontal tissues.
3. Even when the challenges described earlier are overcome, the roots of these teeth are thin with a higher susceptibility to fracture.

These problems are overcome by using a disinfection protocol that does not include root canal instrumentation, stimulating the formation of a hard tissue barrier or providing an artificial apical barrier to allow for optimal filling of the canal, and reinforcing the weakened root against fracture during and after an apical stop is provided.

TRADITIONAL TECHNIQUE
Disinfection of the Canal

Because in most cases nonvital teeth are infected,[1,2] the first phase of treatment is to disinfect the root canal system to ensure periapical healing.[2,3] The canal length is estimated with a parallel preoperative radiograph, and after access to the canal is made, a file is placed to this length. After the length has been confirmed radiographically, depending on the thickness of the remaining dentinal walls either a very light filing or no

---

[a] University of Pennsylvania, Philadelphia, PA 19104, USA
[b] University of North Carolina School of Dentistry, Chapel Hill, NC 27599, USA
* 1601 Walnut Street, Suite 401, Philadelphia, PA 19102.
E-mail address: martintrope@gmail.com

Dent Clin N Am 54 (2010) 313–324
doi:10.1016/j.cden.2009.12.006
dental.theclinics.com

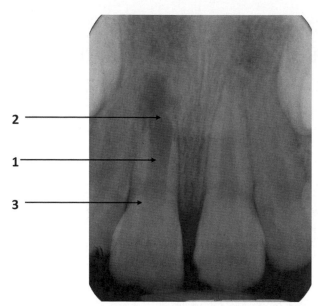

Fig. 1. The immature root with a necrotic pulp and apical periodontitis presents multiple challenges to successful treatment. (1) The infected root canal space cannot be disinfected with the standard root canal protocol with the aggressive use of endodontic files. (2) Once the microbial phase of treatment is complete, filling the root canal is difficult because the open apex provides no barrier for stopping the root filling material before impinging on the periodontal tissues. (3) Even if the challenges described earlier are overcome, the roots of these teeth are thin with a higher-than-normal susceptibility to fracture.

filing is performed with copious irrigation with 0.5% sodium hypochlorite.[4,5] A lower strength of sodium hypochlorite is used because of the danger of placing it through the apex of immature teeth. The lower strength of sodium hypochlorite is compensated by the volume of the irrigant used. An irrigation needle that can passively reach close to the apical length is useful in disinfecting the canals of immature teeth. The intra-canal medication is placed when the irrigant leaving the canal is clean of debris. Newer irrigation protocols such as EndoVac[6] (Discus Dental, Culver City, CA, USA) or use of ultrasound[7] may be useful in immature canals.

The canal is dried with paper points, and a creamy mix of calcium hydroxide is spun into the canal with a lentulospiral instrument. The disinfecting action of calcium hydroxide (in addition to instrumentation and irrigation) is effective after its application for at least 1 week,[8] so that the continuation of treatment can take place any time after 1 week. Further treatment should not be delayed for more than 1 month because the calcium hydroxide could be washed out by tissue fluids through the open apex, leaving the canal susceptible to reinfection.

A new disinfection medicament has been used when revascularization is attempted (discussed in later section). This medicament has been extensively studied by Sato and colleagues[9] and Hoshino and colleagues.[10] It comprises metronidazole, ciprofloxacin, and minocycline in a saline or glycerin vehicle. A recent study by Windley and colleagues[11] showed the effectiveness of the tri-antibiotic paste when used for a month on immature infected dog teeth that had been irrigated with only sodium hypochlorite.

Hard Tissue Apical Barrier

Traditional method

The formation of the hard tissue barrier at the apex requires an environment similar to that required for hard tissue formation in vital pulp therapy, that is a mild inflammatory stimulus to initiate healing and a bacteria-free environment to ensure that the inflammation is not progressive.

As with vital pulp therapy, calcium hydroxide is used for this procedure.[12–14] Pure calcium hydroxide powder is mixed with sterile saline (or anesthetic solution) to a thick (powdery) consistency (**Fig. 2**). Ready mixed commercially available calcium hydroxide can also be used. The calcium hydroxide is packed against the apical soft tissue with a plugger or a thick point to initiate hard tissue formation. This step is followed by backfilling with calcium hydroxide to completely fill the canal thus ensuring a bacteria-free canal with little chance of reinfection during the 6 to 18 months required for the hard tissue formation at the apex. The calcium hydroxide is meticulously removed from the access cavity to the level of the root orifices, and a well-sealing temporary filling is placed. When a radiograph is taken, the canal should seem to have become calcified, indicating that the entire canal has been filled with the calcium hydroxide (**Fig. 3**). Because calcium hydroxide washout is evaluated by its relative radiodensity in the canal, it is prudent to use a calcium hydroxide mixture without the addition of a radiopaque substance such as barium sulfate. These additives do not wash out as readily as calcium hydroxide, so if they are present in the canal, evaluation of washout is not possible.

At 3 months' interval a radiograph is taken to evaluate if a hard tissue barrier has formed and if the calcium hydroxide has washed out of the canal. This is assessed to have occurred if the canal can be seen again radiographically. If calcium hydroxide washout is seen, it is replaced as before. If no washout is evident, it can be left intact for another 3 months. Excessive calcium hydroxide dressing changes should be avoided if possible because the initial toxicity of the material is believed to delay healing.[15]

When completion of a hard tissue barrier is suspected, the calcium hydroxide is washed out of the canal with sodium hypochlorite and a radiograph is taken to evaluate the radiodensity of the apical stop. A file that can easily reach the apex is used to gently probe for a stop at the apex. The canal is filled after the presence of

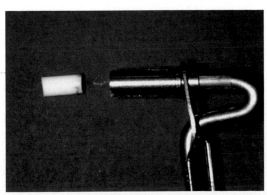

Fig. 2. Pure calcium hydroxide powder mixed with sterile saline (or anesthetic solution) to a thick (powdery) consistency.

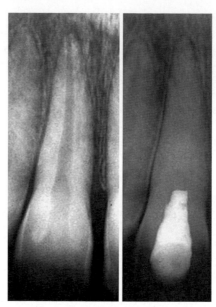

Fig. 3. The canal seems to have become calcified, indicating that the entire canal has been adequately filled with the calcium hydroxide. (*Courtesy of* Frederic Barnett, DMD, Philadelphia, PA.)

a hard tissue barrier is indicated radiographically and the barrier is probed with an instrument.

The hard tissue barrier that forms has been described as "Swiss cheese–like" (**Fig. 4**) because many soft tissue inclusions are still present inside the hard tissue during the time a barrier that can resist a filling material is formed. The soft filling material therefore often passes through the apex in the form of a sealer or filling material puff. The hard tissue barrier is formed at the site of healing of the periodontal granulation tissue. This site does not always conform to the radiographic apex of the tooth. Therefore when the presence of the hard tissue is felt with a point or file, it may be short of the radiographic apex of the tooth. It is important not to force the file to the radiographic apex so as to avoid destruction of the formed barrier.

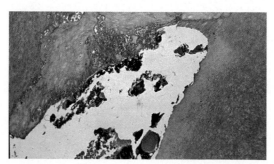

Fig. 4. Histologic appearance of a "Swiss cheese–like" apical hard tissue barrier. Note the soft tissue inclusions inside the hard tissue.

The traditional calcium hydroxide apexification technique has been extensively studied and is proved to have a high success rate.[16,17] However, the technique has some disadvantages. The primary disadvantage is that it typically takes between 6 and 18 months for the body to form the hard tissue barrier. The patient needs to report every 3 months to evaluate whether the calcium hydroxide has washed out and/or the barrier is complete enough to provide a stop to a filling material. This requires patient compliance for up to 6 visits before the procedure is completed. It has also been shown that the use of calcium hydroxide weakens the resistance of the dentin to fracture.[18] Thus it is common for the patient to sustain another injury and also fracture the root before the hard tissue barrier is formed (**Fig. 5**).

Mineral trioxide aggregate barrier

Mineral trioxide aggregate (MTA) is used to create a hard tissue barrier after the disinfection of the canal (**Fig. 6**). Calcium sulfate (or similar material) is pushed through the apex to provide a resorbable extraradicular barrier against which the MTA is packed. The MTA is mixed and placed into the apical 3 to 4 mm of the canal in a manner similar to the placement of calcium hydroxide. A wet cotton pellet can be placed against the MTA and left for at least 6 hours and then the entire canal filled with a root filling material or the filling can be placed immediately because the tissue fluids of the open apex may provide enough moisture to ensure that the MTA sets sufficiently. The cervical canal is then reinforced with composite resin to below the level of the marginal bone as described later in the article (see **Fig. 6**).

Several case reports have been published using this MTA apical barrier technique,[19,20] and it has steadily gained popularity with clinicians. At present, there is no prospective long-term outcome study that compares the success rate of this technique with that of the traditional calcium hydroxide technique.

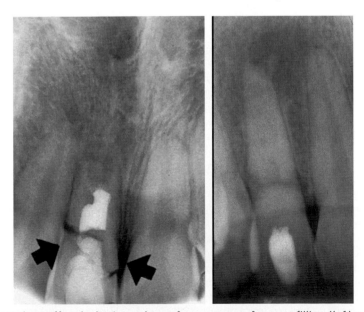

Fig. 5. Root that suffered a horizontal root fracture soon after root filling (*left*) and during the long-term calcium hydroxide treatment (*right*). (*From* Andreasen JO, Farik B, Munksgaard EC. Long-term calcium hydroxide as a root dressing may increase risk of root fracture. Dent Traumatol 2002;18(3):134–7; with permission.)

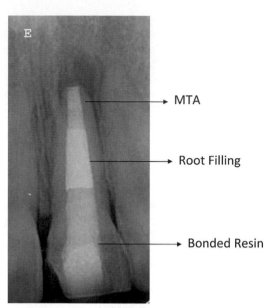

MTA

Root Filling

Bonded Resin

Fig. 6. Apexification with MTA. The canal is disinfected with light instrumentation, copious irrigation, and a creamy mix of calcium hydroxide for 1 month, calcium sulfate is placed through the apex as a barrier to the placement of MTA, and 4-mm MTA plug is placed at the apex. The body of the canal is filled with Resilon obturation system (Pentron Clinical Technologies, Wallingford, CT, USA), and a bonded resin is placed to below the cementoe-namel junction to strengthen the root. (*Courtesy of* Marga Ree, DDS, MSc, Purmerend, Netherlands.)

Because the apical diameter is larger than the coronal diameter of most of the canals, a softened filling technique is indicated for these teeth. Care must be taken to avoid excessive lateral force during filling because of the thin walls of the root.

The apexification procedure has become a predictably successful procedure.[16,17] However, the thin dentinal walls still present a clinical problem. Should secondary injuries occur, teeth with thin dentinal walls are more susceptible to fractures that render them nonrestorable. It has been reported that approximately 30% of these teeth will fracture during or after endodontic treatment (see **Fig. 5**).[16] Some clinicians have there-fore questioned the advisability of the apexification procedure and have opted for more radical treatment procedures, including extraction followed by extensive restorative procedures such as dental implants. Studies have shown that intracoronal bonded restorations can internally strengthen endodontically treated teeth and increase their resistance to fracture.[21,22] Thus after root filling, the material should be removed to below the level of marginal bone and a bonded resin filling placed (see **Fig. 6**).

Routine recall evaluation should be performed to determine the success in the prevention or treatment of apical periodontitis. Restorative procedures should be as-sessed to ensure that they do not promote root fractures.

Periapical healing and the formation of a hard tissue barrier occurs predictably with long-term calcium hydroxide treatment (79%–96%).[14] However, long-term survival is jeopardized by the fracture potential of the thin dentinal walls of these teeth. It is ex-pected that the newer techniques of internally strengthening the teeth described earlier will increase their long-term survivability.

PULP REVASCULARIZATION

Revascularization of a necrotic pulp is considered possible only after avulsion of an immature permanent tooth. Skoglund and colleagues[23] showed in dog teeth that pulp revascularization was possible and took approximately 45 days (**Fig. 7**). The advantages of pulp revascularization lie in the possibility of further root development and reinforcement of dentinal walls by deposition of hard tissue thus strengthening the root against fracture. After reimplantation of an avulsed immature tooth, a unique set of circumstances exists that allows revascularization to take place. The young tooth has an open apex and is short; this allows new tissue to grow into the pulp space quickly. The pulp is necrotic but usually not degenerated and infected; thus it acts as a scaffold into which the new tissue can grow. The apical part of a pulp may remain vital and after reimplantation may proliferate coronally, replacing the necrotized portion of the pulp.[23–26] In most cases, the crown of the tooth is intact and caries-free, ensuring that bacterial penetration into the pulp space through cracks[27] and defects is slow. Thus the race between the new tissue formation and infection of the pulp space favors the new tissue.

Revascularization of the pulp space in a necrotic infected tooth with apical periodontitis has been considered to be impossible. Nygaard Ostby[28] successfully regenerated pulps after vital pulp removal in immature teeth, but he was unsuccessful when the pulp space was infected. However, if the canal is effectively disinfected, a scaffold into which new tissue can grow is provided, and the coronal access is effectively sealed, revascularization should occur as in an avulsed immature tooth.

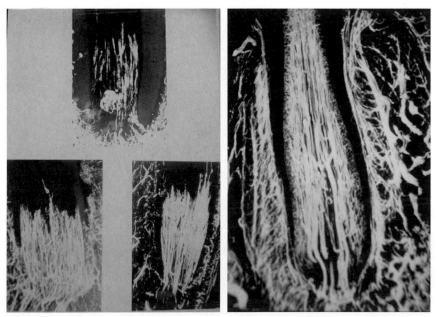

Fig. 7. Revascularization of immature dog teeth during a period of 45 days. The teeth were extracted and immediately replanted. Over the course of 45 days, the blood supply moved into the pulp space. (*From* Skoglund A, Tronstad L, Wallenius K. A microradiographic study of vascular changes in replanted and autotransplanted teeth in young dogs. Oral Surg Oral Med Oral Pathol 1978;45(1):23; with permission.)

A case report by Banchs and Trope[29] has reproduced results in cases reported by others that indicate that it may be possible to replicate the unique circumstances of an avulsed tooth to revascularize the pulp in infected necrotic immature roots.[25,26]

The case (**Fig. 8**) describes the treatment of an immature second lower right premolar tooth with radiographic and clinical signs of apical periodontitis with the presence of a sinus tract. The canal was disinfected without mechanical instrumentation but with copious irrigation with 5.25% sodium hypochlorite and the use of a tri-antibiotic mixture.[9,11]

A blood clot was produced to the level of the cementoenamel junction to provide a scaffold for the ingrowth of new tissue, followed by a double seal of MTA in the cervical area and a bonded resin coronal restoration above it. With clinical and radiographic evidence of healing at 22 days, the large radiolucency had disappeared within 7 months, and at the 24th month recall it was obvious that the root walls were thick and the development of the root below the restoration was similar to the adjacent and contralateral teeth. The author's group has confirmed the potent antibacterial properties of the tri-antibiotic paste used in this case.[11]

Some variations on the original tri-antibiotic paste mixture have been used with good success (**Fig. 9**).[30] These variations were tried because of the staining of the dentin by the antibiotic minocycline (**Fig. 10**). Either the minocycline is left out thus using a bi-antibiotic paste or cefaclor is used as a substitute for the minocycline.[30]

A recent study on dogs demonstrated the potential for revascularization using a collagen-enhanced scaffold (**Fig. 11**). This study also indicated that it was the blood clot with or without the addition of the collagen-enhanced scaffold that seemed important for the stimulation of the revascularization process.[31] The study also confirmed

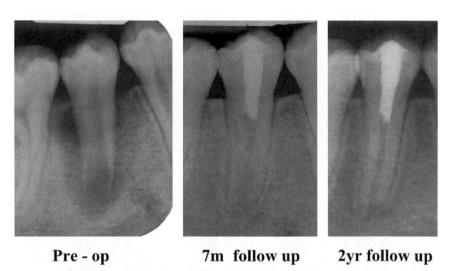

Pre - op   7m follow up   2yr follow up

Fig. 8. Immature tooth with a necrotic infected canal with apical periodontitis. The canal is disinfected with copious irrigation with sodium hypochlorite and tri-antibiotic paste. After 4 weeks the antibiotic is removed, and a blood clot created in the canal space. The access is filled with an MTA base, and bonded resin above it. At 7 months the patient is asymptomatic, and the apex shows healing the apical periodontitis and some closure of the apex. At 24 months apical healing is obvious, and root wall thickening and root lengthening have occurred, indicating that the root canal has been revascularized with vital tissue. (*Adapted from* Banchs F, Trope M. Revascularization of immature permanent teeth with apical periodontitis: new treatment protocol? J Endod 2004;30:196; with permission.)

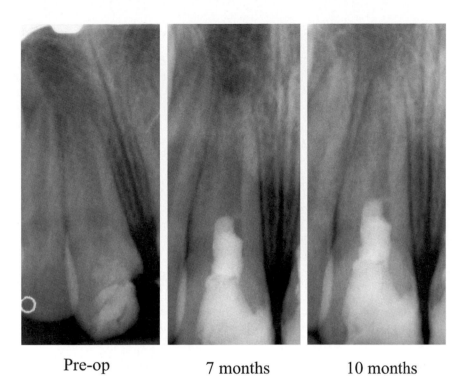

Pre-op   7 months   10 months

Fig. 9. Successful revascularization after failed Cvek pulpotomy. Cefaclor was substituted for minocycline in the tri-antibiotic paste. (*Courtesy of* Blayne Thibodeau, DMD, Saskatoon, Canada.)

that only in a few cases the pulp is actually the tissue that revascularizes the pulp space (see **Fig. 11**). Case-based studies have confirmed the viability of this procedure.[32,33] Further studies are underway to find other potential synthetic matrices that will act as a more predictable scaffold for new ingrowth of tissue than the blood

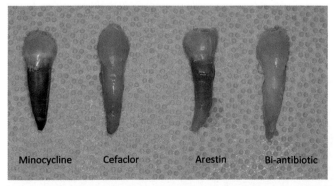

Fig. 10. Discoloration after antibiotic placement. Minocycline in the tri-antibiotic paste seems to be the cause of the discoloration. The color of the root after placement of the paste including minocycline is shown (*first from left*). If Arestin (OraPharma, Inc, Warminster, PA, USA) is used as a substitute for the minocycline, the discoloration is markedly reduced (*third from left*). However cefaclor (*second from left*) or no additional antibiotic (*extreme right*) results in the least discoloration. (*Courtesy of* Dr Jared Buck, Philadelphia, PA.)

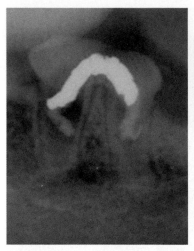 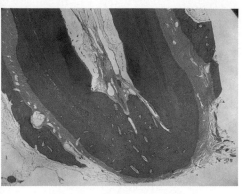

Fig. 11. Experimental confirmation that revascularization is possible. Radiograph on the left is after successful revascularization and root wall thickening. The histologic picture on the right shows cementum on the inner root wall, which is the reason for the thickening of the root. (*From* Thibodeau B, Teixeira F, Yamauchi M, et al. Pulp revascularization of imma-ture dog teeth with apical periodontitis. J Endod 2007;33(6):680–9; with permission.)

clot that was used in previous cases. In addition, a synthetic matrix may allow easier and more predictable placement of the coronal seal than that provided by a fresh blood clot. The procedure described in this section can be attempted in most cases, and if after 3 months no signs of regeneration are present, the more traditional treatment methods can be initiated.

DISCUSSION POINTS
Regeneration Versus Revascularization

Cases such as those presented in this article have been described as examples of pulp regeneration and the beginning of stem cell technology in endodontics. It is important to distinguish between revascularization and pulp regeneration. At present, it is certain that the pulp space has returned to a vital state, but based on research in avulsed teeth and on a recent study on infected teeth, it is likely that the tissue in the pulp space is more similar to periodontal ligament than to pulp tissue (see **Fig. 11**).[31] It seems that there is about a 30% chance of pulp tissue reentering the pulp space.[34] Future research will be needed to stimulate pulp regeneration from the pluripotential cells in the periapical region. Also, in an irreversible pulpitis case, instead of removing the entire pulp and replacing it with a synthetic filling material, partial resection of the pulp and regrowth with the help of a synthetic scaffold would be better.

REFERENCES

1. Bergenholtz G. Micro-organisms from necrotic pulps of traumatized teeth. Odon-tol Revy 1974;25:347–58.
2. Shuping G, Ørstavik D, Sigurdsson A, et al. Reduction of intracanal bacteria using Nickel-titanium rotary instrumentation and various medications. J Endod 2000;26:751–5.

3. Cvek M, Hollender L, Nord CE. Treatment of non-vital permanent incisors with calcium hydroxide. VI. A clinical, microbiological and radiological evaluation of treatment in one sitting of teeth with mature or immature root. Odontol Revy 1976; 27:93.

4. Cvek M, Nord CE, Hollender L. Antimicrobial effect of root canal debridement in teeth with immature root. A clinical and microbiologic study. Odontol Revy 1976; 27(1):1–10.

5. Spangberg L, Rutberg M, Rydinge E. Biologic effects of endodontic antimicrobial agents. J Endod 1979;5:166.

6. Nielsen BA, Craig Baumgartner J. Comparison of the EndoVac system to needle irrigation of root canals. J Endod 2007;33(5):611–5.

7. Carver K, Nusstein J, Reader A, et al. In vivo antibacterial efficacy of ultrasound after hand and rotary instrumentation in human mandibular molars. J Endod 2007;33(9):1038–43.

8. Bystrom A, Claesson R, Sundqvist G. The antibacterial effect of camphorated paramonochlorophenol, camphorated phenol and calcium hydroxide in the treatment of infected root canals. Endod Dent Traumatol 1985;1:170.

9. Sato T, Hoshino E, Uematsu H, et al. In-vitro anti-microbial susceptibility to combinations of drugs on bacteria from carious and endodontic lesions of human deciduous teeth. Oral Microbiol Immunol 1993;8:172–6.

10. Hoshino E, Kurihara-Ando N, Sato I, et al. In-vitro antibacterial susceptibility of bacteria taken from infected root dentine to a mixture of ciprofloxacin, metronidazole and minocycline. Int Endod J 1996;29:125–30.

11. Windley W 3rd, Teixeira F, Levin L, et al. Disinfection of immature teeth with a triple antibiotic paste. J Endod 2005;31(6):439–43.

12. Heithersay GS. Calcium hydroxide in the treatment of pulpless teeth with associated pathology. J Br Endod Soc 1962;8:74.

13. Herforth A, Strassburg M. [Therapy of chronic apical periodontitis in traumatically injuring front teeth with ongoing root growth]. Dtsch Zahnarztl Z 1977;32:453 [in German].

14. Cvek M. Prognosis of luxated non-vital maxillary incisors treated with calcium hydroxide and filled with gutta-percha. A retrospective clinical study. Endod Dent Traumatol 1992;8:45.

15. Lengheden A, Blomlof L, Lindskog S. Effect of delayed calcium hydroxide treatment on periodontal healing in contaminated replanted teeth. Scand J Dent Res 1991;99:147.

16. Kerekes K, Heide S, Jacobsen I. Follow-up examination of endodontic treatment in traumatized juvenile incisors. J Endod 1980;6(9):744–8.

17. Frank AL. Therapy for the divergent pulpless tooth by continued apical formation. J Am Dent Assoc 1966;72:87.

18. Andreasen JO, Farik B, Munksgaard EC. Long-term calcium hydroxide as a root canal dressing may increase risk of root fracture. Dent Traumatol 2002;18:134.

19. Giuliani V, Baccetti T, Pace R, et al. The use of MTA in teeth with necrotic pulps and open apices. Dent Traumatol 2002;18:217.

20. Maroto M, Barberia E, Planells P, et al. Treatment of a non-vital immature incisor with mineral trioxide aggregate (MTA). Dent Traumatol 2003;19:165.

21. Katebzadeh N, Dalton BC, Trope M. Strengthening immature teeth during and after apexification. J Endod 1998;24:256.

22. Goldberg F, Kaplan A, Roitman M, et al. Reinforcing effect of a resin glass ionomer in the restoration of immature roots in vitro. Dent Traumatol 2002; 18:70.

23. Skoglund A, Tronstad L, Wallenius K. A microradiographic study of vascular changes in replanted and autotransplanted teeth in young dogs. Oral Surg Oral Med Oral Pathol 1978;45(1):172–8.
24. Barrett AP, Reade PC. Revascularization of mouse tooth isografts and allografts using autoradiography and carbon-perfusion. Arch Oral Biol 1981;26:541.
25. Rule DC, Winter GB. Root growth and apical repair subsequent to pulpal necrosis in children. Braz Dent J 1966;120:586–90.
26. Iwaya SI, Ikawa M, Kubota M. Revascularization of an immature permanent tooth with apical periodontitis and sinus tract. Dent Traumatol 2001;17:185–7.
27. Love RM. Bacterial penetration of the root canal of intact incisor teeth after a simulated traumatic injury. Endod Dent Traumatol 1996;12:289.
28. Nygaard-Ostby B, Hjortdal O, Murrah V, et al. Tissue formation in the root canal following pulp removal. Scand J Dent Res 1971;79:333–49.
29. Banchs F, Trope M. Revascularization of immature permanent teeth with apical periodontitis: new treatment protocol? J Endod 2004;30:196.
30. Thibodeau B, Trope M. Pulp revascularization of a necrotic infected immature permanent tooth: case report and review of the literature. Pediatr Dent 2007; 29:47.
31. Thibodeau B, Teixeira F, Yamauchi M, et al. Pulp revascularization of immature dog teeth with apical periodontitis. J Endod 2007;33(6):680–9.
32. Jung IY, Lee SJ, Hargreaves JM. Biologically based treatment of immature permanent teeth with pulpal necrosis: a case series. J Endod 2008;7:876.
33. Bose R, Nummikoski P, Hargreaves K. A retrospective evaluation of radiographic outcomes in immature teeth with necrotic root canal systems treated with regenerative endodontic procedures. J Endod 2009;10:1343.
34. Ritter AL, Ritter AV, Murrah V, et al. Pulp revascularization of replanted immature dog teeth after treatment with minocycline and doxycycline assessed by laser Doppler flowmetry, radiography, and histology. Dent Traumatol 2004;20:75–84.

Resin Materials for Root Canal Obturation

Cornelis H. Pameijer, DMD, MScD, DSc, PhD[a,b,]*,
Osvaldo Zmener, DDS, Dr Odont[c]

KEYWORDS

- Methacrylate resins • Obturation • Biocompatibility
- Leakage • Cytotoxicity

DEVELOPMENT LEADING TO RESIN SEALERS

The concept of resin bonding in dentistry was introduced in the mid-1950s by Buono-core,[1] who advocated the use of an acid to demineralize enamel. Skepticism slowly gave way to general acceptance. However, bonding materials and techniques have completely changed over the course of 50 years. During the initial development only hydrophobic resins were available; these have been replaced by hydrophilic resins over time. Furthermore, about 30 years of research resulted in a change from using 85% phosphoric acid liquid for 60 seconds to etch enamel to 35% phosphoric acid gels for 15 seconds to etch dentin and enamel. Although early attempts were strictly focused on preventive and restorative dentistry, it was only a matter of time before orthodontics and then endodontics embraced this concept. Usually, when new materials and techniques are introduced, there is an initial reluctance on the part of practitioners to abandon trusted and proven methods until evidence that is sufficiently convincing to change established techniques is generated.

The objective of this article is to provide information about methacrylate-based resin sealers (MBRS) on which practitioners can base their decision to consider changing established techniques and embrace a new one. This decision cannot be made by presenting empiric data, but by offering an analysis of scientific evidence from ex vivo and in vivo research. Based on their successful long-track record, gutta-percha and zinc oxide, eugenol, and other conventional sealers, have served as the gold standard for comparison.

[a] Department of Reconstructive Sciences, University of Connecticut, Health Center, Farmington, CT 06030, USA
[b] DLC International, 10 Highwood, Simsbury CT 06070, USA
[c] Post Graduate Program for Specialized Endodontics, Faculty of Medical Sciences, School of Dentistry, University of El Salvador, Buenos Aires, Argentina
* Corresponding author. Department of Reconstructive Sciences, University of Connecticut, Health Center, Farmington, CT 06030.
E-mail address: cornelis@pameijer.com

Dent Clin N Am 54 (2010) 325–344
doi:10.1016/j.cden.2009.12.004
0011-8532/10/$ – see front matter © 2010 Elsevier Inc. All rights reserved.

dental.theclinics.com

One of the factors that was instrumental in the development of resin-based sealers was the recognition that gutta-percha does not bond to dentin or to any conventionally used sealer, such as zinc oxide-eugenol (ZOE)-based cements and epoxy resins such as AH-26 or AH Plus. Although these materials are being used successfully, an ideal root canal sealer should be capable of bonding to root canal dentin and to gutta-percha, thus preventing microleakage. Recent advances in adhesive technology have led to the introduction of a new generation of endodontic sealers and filling materials, that are based on adhesive properties and polymer resin technology. These materials are capable of forming a hybrid layer and penetrating deep into dentinal tubules by virtue of their hydrophilic properties.

Early attempts at using resins were reported in 1978 by Tidmarsh,[2] who suggested that a low-viscosity resin could have the potential to be used in root canal obturation. Of the bonding agents that were used in restorative dentistry, the early generations did not use an acid to remove the smear layer and therefore bonded to it. This resulted in a weak bond and did not prevent bacterial leakage. Later generations that used 35% phosphoric acid gels for the removal of the smear layer were more promising. Furthermore, the early resins were hydrophobic and therefore their interaction was adversely affected by moisture in the dentin. The latest bonding agents are hydrophilic and they derive their adhesive properties from micromechanical interlocking by penetrating into dentinal tubules, thus creating an attachment mechanism along with an intimate hybrid layer when they come in direct contact with the surrounding collagen fibrillar intertubular network. The latter requires careful treatment and it has been shown that the collagen network of dentin can be best preserved using 17% to 19% EDTA[3] or low concentrations of citric acid solution as the final rinse. Effective removal of the smear layer before filling the canals will enhance the ability of these bonding agents to enter the dentinal tubules and improve the sealing of the root canal system by increasing the contact surface area. The presence of organic debris along with bacteria within the matrix of the smear layer represents an undesirable interface between filling material and dentin. Furthermore, the sequence of the irrigating solutions has been shown to be a factor. A 5% sodium hypochlorite (NaOCl) solution followed by 17% EDTA or 50% citric acid seems to be the most effective combination.[4,5]

Zidan and El Deeb[6] were among the first to attempt to establish adhesion to dentin walls in vitro with the use of Scotchbond (3M ESPE, St Paul, MN, USA). Apical microleakage with gutta-percha and the bonding agent was significantly less than in root canals obturated with gutta-percha and Tubli-Seal (SybronEndo, West Collins, Orange, CA, USA), a ZOE-based root canal sealer. Handling properties, radiopacity, and the difficulty of removing the sealer in case of retreatment were some of the drawbacks that were experienced. Other possible bonding systems have subsequently been reported in the literature. Leonard and colleagues[7] compared the effectiveness of a combination of the dentin bonding agent 4-methacryloyloxyethy trimellitate anhydride (4-META) and the resin C&B Metabond (Parkell Inc, Edgewood, NY, USA), which was commercialized a few years later as MetaSEAL (Parkell Inc, Edgewood, NY, USA), and the glass ionomer cement Ketac-Endo (3M ESPE, St Paul, MN, USA) for sealing of the root canal system. The coronal and apical seals were tested by means of dye penetration, and both materials showed some evidence of dye leakage. However, the sealing ability of the bonding agent and resin was significantly better. This was further supported by scanning electron microscopy (SEM) of the interface sealer and dentin, indicating the presence of a hybrid layer and resin tags penetrating into the dentinal tubules. Despite these positive features, the materials seemed to be technique sensitive. Nikaido and colleagues,[8] Morris and colleagues,[9] and Erdemir and colleagues,[10] showed that the use of sodium hypochlorite and hydrogen peroxide or a combination of both irrigants, decreased the bond strength to dentin by adversely affecting the tensile bond strength to bovine dentin. Hydrogen peroxide breaks down to water and oxygen, whereas the combination of sodium hypochlorite and hydrogen peroxide allows for the formation of oxygen, which inhibits polymerization of the adhesive materials. However, irrigation with chlorhexidine did not exhibit these adverse effects.

ALL-BOND 2 adhesive (Bisco, Itasca, IL) and Scotchbond Multi-purpose Plus adhesive in combination with gutta-percha and an epoxy resin–based root canal sealer AH-26 (Dentsply-Maillefer, Switzerland) was also tested for leakage with a 2% methylene blue solution.[11] It was reported that root canals that had the combination of bonding agents with gutta-percha and the epoxy resin sealer leaked significantly less than the controls in which the root canals were obturated with gutta-percha and AH-26. Although no problems were experienced with respect to the working time of the bonding agents, the complexity of the technique (it required many steps) made the use of bonding agents impractical for root canal obturation. Of additional concern is the use of bonding agents containing 2-hydroxyethyl methacrylate (HEMA), which, when extruded beyond the apex into bone, could sensitize patients, particularly if they are from Nordic countries or have genetic make-up that originates there.

Ahlberg and Tay[12] tested a methacrylate-based bone cement normally used in orthopedic surgery, in which the monomer from N-butyl methacrylate was changed to tetrahydrofurfuryl methacrylate with 1% N'N'-dimethyl p-toluidine as the activator. The powder consisted of poly(ethyl methacrylate) with a molecular weight of 150,000 to 1,500,000 and a particle size of 15 to 100 μm. They used this formulation to obturate in vitro root canals of human teeth with gutta-percha cones; the control canals were filled with gutta-percha only. The root canals filled with the resin and gutta-percha leaked significantly less than the controls. Scanning electron microscope observation of the interface revealed a bond not only between the resin-based sealer and the root canal walls but also between the sealer and gutta-percha. With respect to their handling properties, the material was found to be easy to place in the root canal and the working time was approximately 50 minutes. The investigators postulated that, because the smear layer was not effectively removed, bonding to the root canal walls may be attributed to the low viscosity of the resin itself, whereas the ability to bond to gutta-percha was attributed to dissolution of the gutta-percha surface.

Kataoka and colleagues[13] analyzed the coronal and apical sealing properties of a newly developed resin-based root canal sealer composed of vinylidine fluoride/hexafluoropropylene copolymer, methyl methacrylate, zirconia, and tributylborane as the catalyst, used in conjunction with gutta-percha cones in root canals, which were pretreated with dentin conditioners and primers. They also analyzed the tensile bond strength and used SEM to analyze the interfaces. The test material revealed a significantly higher sealing ability than Pulp Canal Sealer EWT (Sybron Kerr, Romulus, MI, USA) and Sealapex (Sybron Kerr, Romulus, MI, USA), which were used as controls. When the canal walls were pretreated with EDTA and further application of glutaraldehyde/2-hydroxyethyl methacrylate primers, higher bond strength values were recorded. SEM observation revealed the presence of a hybrid layer approximately 2 μm thick, formed by the penetration of the resin into the dentin with only a few gaps at the interface between the sealer and the root canal walls. Based on these observations, the investigators suggested that the tested resin-based sealer had many useful properties for root canal obturation, such as adhesiveness to dentin and gutta-percha while exhibiting good sealing properties.

According to the above information these experimental formulations have the potential to bond to the root canal walls provided the smear layer is removed.

METHACRYLATE-BASED RESIN SEALERS

MBRS are new in endodontics and are derived from polymer chemistry technology initially developed for adhesive restorative dentistry, albeit in modified formulations and viscosities as determined by the specific demands in endodontics. This article focuses on 2 systems as they dominate the market:

1. EndoREZ (Ultradent Products Inc, South Jordan, UT, USA) and
2. RealSeal (Sybron Dental Specialties, Orange, CA, USA).

Pentron Clinical Technologies (Wallingford, CT, USA) was recently acquired by Sybron Dental Specialties, which includes the Resilon-Epiphany system, now marketed as RealSeal. Therefore products such as SimpliFill (LightSpeed Technology Inc, San Antonio, TX, USA), InnoEndo (Heraeus Kulzer, Armonk, NJ, USA), and Resinate (Obtura Spartan, Fenton, MO, USA) and Resilon-Epiphany are now all categorized under the name RealSeal.

ENDOREZ

EndoREZ (ER) is a hydrophilic, two-component (base and catalysts), dual-curing self-priming sealer. The formulation can be described as follows:

The EndoREZ base contains:
    a bismuth compound as the radiopaque filler
    small amounts of other fillers
    diurethane dimethacrylate
    triethylene glycol dimethacrylate
    a peroxide initiator
    a photo initiator (not chamfer quinone).
The EndoREZ catalyst contains:
    a bismuth compound as the radiopaque filler
    small amounts of other fillers
    diurethane dimethacrylate
    triethylene glycol dimethacrylate.

The sealer can be used with gutta-percha or with resin-coated gutta-percha cones, the latter with the objective of establishing continuous adhesion (uniblock or monobloc) between all materials. The sealer is supplied in a double barrel auto mixing and delivery syringe and meets the basic requirements of an endodontic sealer. The manufacturer recommends that after preparation the root canal walls should remain slightly moist to take maximum advantage of the hydrophilic properties of the sealer, thus allowing for resin tags to penetrate into the dentinal tubules and the formation of a hybrid layer with the collagen fiber network.[14] However, too much water can cause water permeation during the polymerization process and results in the entrapment of water droplets in the sealer, resulting in bond disruption and an increase in leakage.[15] Delivery through the tiny opening and the hydraulics involved when using a NaviTip (Ultradent Products Inc, South Jordan, UT, USA) produces a sealer free from air bubbles that fills the canal with a homogeneous layer. The sealer is radiopaque and has favorable low viscosity properties. Low viscosity plays a significant role in the handling properties and makes it useful for placement in wide or narrow root canals; it provides a good adaptation to the intricacies of the dentin walls. EndoREZ bonds well to root canal walls but not to gutta-percha, which constitutes a potential weakness, as a path for bacterial leakage may exist.[16] To address this issue and to establish a bond between sealer and dentin and between sealer and gutta-percha, resin-coated gutta-percha cones (RCGP) cones (Ultradent Products Inc, South Jordan, UT, USA) were introduced.

The combination of these materials establishes the so-called monobloc and is the reason for the superior sealing properties of the system. The objective of the EndoREZ sealer is to establish a hermetic seal, rather than high bond strength adhesion, that is, optimum softness or hardness while providing a maximum seal.

The RCGP cones can be used with an accelerator, which serves a dual purpose. The polymerization reaction of the EndoREZ is accelerated (within 4–5 minutes) allowing for immediate continuation of the restorative phase should the practitioner choose to do so and bonding of the EndoREZ to the RCGP cones is promoted, thus establishing a monobloc.

REALSEAL (RESILON/EPIPHANY)

Resilon is composed of a polymer-based resin (polycaprolactone), bioactive glass, bismuth oxide, barium sulfate and coloring agents. The sealer is a dual-cure sealer, composed of urethane dimethacrylate (UDMA), poly dimethacrylate (PEGDMA), ethoxylated bisphenol A dimethacrylate (EBPADMA) and bisphenol A glycidyl methacrylate (BIS-GMA), barium borosilicate, barium sulfate ($BaSO_4$), bismuth oxychloride, calcium hydroxide, photo initiators, and a thinning resin. In addition the system comes with a self-etching primer. The premise behind the material is the formation of a monobloc, that is, the primer forms a hybrid layer with dentin, which bonds to sealer, and then bonds to the Resilon core. The ability of Resilon to bond to methacrylate-based root canal sealers has also been questioned because the amount of dimethacrylate in the thermoplastic composite may not be optimum for chemical coupling.[17] However, when surface roughness was established, the micromechanical interlocking increased the mean bond strength significantly.

BIOCOMPATIBILITY

Several early publications (2001 and 2003) have reported on the biocompatibility and adhesiveness of EndoREZ.[18–20] Since then numerous publications have appeared, testing different MBRS formulations and using a variety of techniques, which to a large extent have caused more controversy and confusion than answering the following basic questions:

1. Are resin-based sealers safe?
2. Can they be used successfully in patients?
3. Will they ultimately replace gutta-percha and conventional sealers?
4. Will they last as long as conventional materials?
5. Are they easier to use than conventional materials?

TOXICOLOGY STUDIES IN VITRO

One of the requirements of any dental material for use in humans is that it should be biocompatible. Numerous investigators have conducted cytotoxicity studies ex vivo using cell cultures and in vivo in laboratory animals. The results between investigators are contradictory. Huang and colleagues[21] showed that the elution compounds from MBRS, zinc oxide-eugenol and calcium hydroxide-based sealers were cytotoxic to primary human periodontal ligament cultures and V79 cells, with calcium hydroxide being the least toxic. Huang and co-workers,[22] reported that the highest level of

DNA damage was induced by epoxy resin–based sealers, in this case Topseal (Dentsply, Konstanz, Switzerland), AH-26, and AH Plus. Koulaouzidou and colleagues[23] reported similar results. AH-26 had a severe cytotoxic effect, whereas Topseal and AH Plus had markedly lower effects. These findings are surprising as the basic formulation of AH-26 and Topseal is the same. Bouillaguet and colleagues,[24] reported that: "Most materials pose significant cytotoxic risks and that cytotoxicity generally decreased with time." At 72 hours, GuttaFlow became significantly less toxic than AH Plus, Epiphany sealer, and Resilon. Other investigators, such as Key and colleagues[25] found Epiphany to be less toxic than Grossman's sealer. However, Epiphany was more cytotoxic than Sealapex after 1 hour, but less after 24 hours. Epiphany was more cytotoxic than conventional materials. In a more recent publication[26] similar findings were reported. According to Lodiene and colleagues[27] the multi-methacrylate-based resin (Epiphany) root canal sealer was significantly more toxic to L-929 cells than the silicone-based RoekoSeal and the single methacrylate-based EndoREZ root canal sealers. AH Plus showed intermediate toxicity.

Based on the these findings it seems that no sealer is universally accepted as being nontoxic. Furthermore, the investigators mentioned earlier have reported completely opposite findings, which makes selection of a sealer without drawbacks difficult, if not impossible. Therefore it is necessary to conduct a careful and critical analysis of the various ex vivo research methodologies to reach a consensus. It is also important to correlate the results of the various techniques with the clinical performance of the same material or materials. Oliver and Abbott[28] reported that clinical and in vitro data frequently contradict each other.

TOXICOLOGY STUDIES IN VIVO

The early studies on which the launch of EndoREZ was based were conducted by Louw and colleagues[18] and Becce and Pameijer[20] who reported that EndoREZ was mildly irritating, but within acceptable standards (1.5° is the acceptable limit). Further evidence of biocompatibility was published by Zmener[29] and Zmener and colleagues.[30] In other related studies (Pameijer, 2002, unpublished data), EndoREZ and Epiphany/Resilon reacted more favorably than the control AH Plus. Preoperative and postoperative radiographs were made and root canal treatment was performed according to a standardized protocol using a rubber dam in subhuman primates. Histologic observations were made at various time periods: 30 days to determine an early reaction and from 3 months to 6 months posttreatment for long-term reactions. The results can be summarized as follows. Ten EndoREZ root canal treated teeth scored a mean inflammatory reaction after 26 days of 1.5°. After 90 days, out of 21 root fills, 4 had extruded sealer with an inflammatory mean of 0.8°. Good apical adaptation scored a lower mean inflammation of 0.4°. None of the periapical areas of the roots at either time period showed bone resorption. The control sealer (AH Plus) had a mean inflammatory reaction of 1.3° after 26 days and 1.0° after 90 days. Epiphany, which was tested according to the same protocol, scored a mean inflammatory reaction of all root fills of 1.2° after 120 days (13 teeth), whereas the inflammation of bone was 0.4°. Control teeth (AH Plus) had a mean inflammatory reaction of 2°, and a bone inflammation of 1°.

Both materials clearly reacted more favorably than the control AH Plus.

These results were confirmed by Zmener.[29] The severity of the reaction decreased over time. Zmener and colleagues[30] conducted a histologic and histometric study in which silicone tubes filled with EndoREZ were implanted in the tibias of rats for a period of 10 days and 60 days. At the 10-day observation period, the number of inflammatory cells in contact with the sealer was significantly higher. After 60 days, the initial inflammatory reaction was resolved and newly formed healthy bone was observed surrounding the implants. Thus, after early mild irritation the material reacted in a biocompatible fashion allowing healing of bone. In contrast Sousa and colleagues[31] tested AH Plus, EndoREZ, and Epiphany in guinea pigs over 4 and 12 weeks. They reported a severe reaction for EndoREZ; AH Plus was also severe after 4 weeks and moderate after 12 weeks. Only Epiphany showed intraosseous biocompatibility.

EXAMPLES OF SEALER AND POINT BIOCOMPATIBILITY TESTING

The periapical tissues can react to extrusion of a sealer and/or point in several ways:

1. It can cause an inflammatory reaction
2. It can be regarded as a foreign body and be encapsulated
3. A sealer can be present without causing inflammatory reactions and is not encapsulated
4. The sealer can be resorbed over time, with or without an inflammatory reaction.

As mentioned earlier, a material causing an inflammatory reaction is not necessarily bad and the outcome depends on the intensity and duration of the inflammatory process and the ability of the natural defense mechanisms of the body to manage the reaction. Biocompatibility should be construed in a broader sense. If over a reasonable period of time (30–60 days) healing occurs after an initial irritating reaction, a material can still be considered biocompatible. None of the endodontic sealers that are currently being used are totally nonirritating, yet without doubt they are being used with clinical success.

If over a short period of time (up to 30 days) a mild inflammation is present and it diminishes over time, a material with otherwise favorable properties can be considered biocompatible.[29] Eluation of components was recognized by Ferracane and Condon[32] and the inflammatory process as a result of this is the body's response to irritation. Fibrous encapsulation without inflammation is the body's response to isolate an otherwise biocompatible material. Furthermore, a material, usually small size particles, can be present in periapical tissues, cause no inflammation, and be present without encapsulation.

Fig. 1 is a representative radiograph of experimental sealers in 4 central incisors. After 113 days 2 reactions were observed for 2 different experimental sealers. **Fig. 2** is an example of extrusion (intentional to determine biocompatibility) of the sealer into periapical tissues. The sealer particles are not encapsulated and no inflammatory reaction was observed. The periapical tissues reacted differently to the other sealer. After 113 days the histologic features of the apical area (**Fig. 3**) showed slight extrusion into the periapical tissues. A fibrous encapsulation of the material can be observed, however, without the presence of inflammatory cells (magnification ×64, hematoxylin and eosin stain).

LEAKAGE STUDIES

Leakage of MBRS, whether coronal or apical, has been studied by numerous investigators, resulting in the publication of contradictory data that have generated more questions than answers.

It has been established that selection of an appropriate sealer will influence the outcome of endodontic therapy.[33,34] For that reason many investigators have focused on this important aspect using techniques such as fluid filtration, dye penetration, and

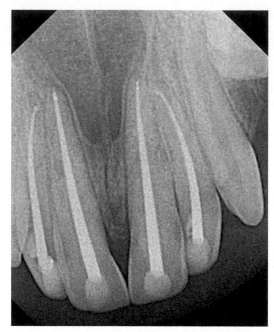

Fig. 1. At 113 days post treatment, the endodontic radiograph of 4 central incisors shows extrusion of sealer (intentional) into the periapical tissues.

bacterial leakage tests. Frequently AH Plus or AH-26 are used as control materials. In one of the first published leakage tests using India ink, Zmener and Banegas[35] reported no statistically significant difference between EndoREZ and AH Plus. Orucoglu and colleagues,[36] using the fluid filtration method, reported that Diaket with cold lateral condensation leaked less apically than EndoREZ and AH Plus. However,

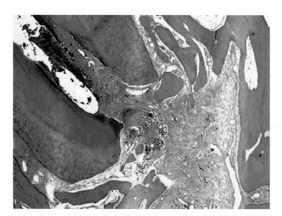

Fig. 2. Histologic reaction of an experimental sealer (*black*) extruded into periapical tissues. The white space was occupied by the Resilon point and disappeared during processing for histology. Ingrowth of connective tissue into apical root space adjacent to the point can be observed. Despite the presence of numerous sealer particles beyond the apex, no inflammatory cells were present (hematoxylin and eosin stain, original magnification ×64).

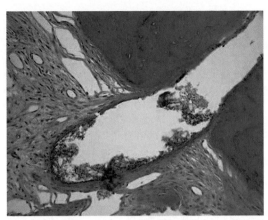

Fig. 3. At 113 days post endodontic treatment, the sealer (*dark brown*) is surrounded by a fibrous capsule in the periodontal ligament space. No inflammatory reaction is present as a result of the extruded material, point, and sealer (hematoxylin and eosin stain, original magnification ×200).

others[37] reported that AH Plus leaked less than EndoREZ and AH-26 using a single cone technique. Compared with zinc oxide-eugenol,[38] MBRS was found to be more effective in sealing. These investigators also used the fluid filtration method. Using similar techniques,[39] it was found that the apical seal of Epiphany and Resilon was not different from AH Plus and gutta-percha, AH Plus and Resilon, and Epiphany and gutta-percha. In contrast, using a fluid-transport method, Tunga and Bodrumlu[40] concluded that Epiphany and Resilon leaked significantly less ($P<.05$) than gutta-percha and AH-26. Others reached a similar conclusion when comparing Resilon and gutta-percha and AH Plus,[41] and in bacterial leakage tests[42,43]; Epiphany and Resilon were superior to gutta-percha and various other sealers. Pitout and colleagues[44] also used a bacterial leakage test and a dye penetration method and Biggs and colleagues[45] did not observe a difference between Resilon and gutta-percha. Several investigators have used the dye penetration technique to demonstrate that MBRSs are superior or inferior to conventional materials.[46–48] One explanation for the difference in results between the various MBRS materials can most likely be attributed to the presence or absence of moisture in the root canal at the time of obturation.

To put leakage studies in context, in 2001 Oliver and Abbott[28] conducted a study to determine if there was a correlation between apical dye penetration and clinical performance of root fillings. They tested the length of apical dye penetration using a vacuum technique ex vivo in 116 human roots that had been root-filled at least 6 months before extraction. Endodontic treatment was classified as clinically successful or unsuccessful and the results for these groups were compared using an analysis of variance and the Student t-test. Positive and negative controls were used to test the experimental system. In unsuccessful cases the dye penetrated significantly further although the raw data suggested little difference. Overall, the dye penetrated in 99.5% of the specimens, and this indicates that the presence of dye in a canal is a poor indicator of whether a technique or material will succeed clinically. However, the extent of dye penetration may be related to the clinical outcome. The investigators concluded that clinically placed root canal fillings do not provide an apical seal that prevents fluid penetration and therefore the outcome of treatment cannot be predicted based on the results of apical dye leakage studies. In 1993 Wu and Wesselink[49] reviewed the shortcomings of various tests reported in the literature. However, dye leakage studies may be useful to determine the performance of a new material or technique by conducting comparative studies with existing systems. An electrochemical technique that seems to be sensitive and has generated findings that correlate with bacterial leakage tests, has been published by von Fraunhofer and colleagues.[50] **Fig. 4** illustrates a comparison between resin sealers and conventional sealers.

Independent of the technique used (fluid filtration or bacterial leakage test or other tests), there is no general agreement on whether there is reduced or more leakage when using MBRS. In addition ex vivo tests frequently do not correlate with clinical performance.

WHEN TO DRY AND WHEN NOT TO DRY

The contradictory data of several of the leakage studies can be explained and are most likely the result of the ingrained belief in endodontics that root canals after a final rinse need to be dried thoroughly. Many articles reviewed stated in the materials and methods section that "the canals were dried" (eg, Biggs and colleagues[45] and Kardon and colleagues[51]). Several of the articles did not specify in sufficient detail the condition of the root canal. Based on established endodontic techniques we can speculate with a fair amount of certainty that the canals were thoroughly dried. Thorough drying will create a hydrophobic environment while a hydrophilic material is being used. Field emission scanning electron microscopy (FESEM) and SEM have provided excellent examples of the potential of EndoREZ when proper moist conditions are adhered to and the recommended insertion technique is followed (**Fig. 5**) and show what happens when the canal is thoroughly dried according to well-established endodontic techniques (**Fig. 6**). The concept of moist bonding has always been difficult to explain in restorative dentistry, and endodontics has not been exempt from the same misinterpretations and misconceptions. For MBRS, whether EndoREZ or Epiphany, to establish a proper seal, the dentin needs to be moist to allow for the penetration of resin tags into the opened dentinal tubules and the formation of a hybrid layer, thus taking advantage of the hydrophilicity of these materials, whether bonding agent or sealer. In the case of EndoREZ this allows for deep penetration of resin tags, up to 500 to 1000 μm and more, and for Epiphany it allows bonding of the adhesive by means of a hybrid layer and resin tags into the dentin. Unlike restorative dentistry, where a reflection

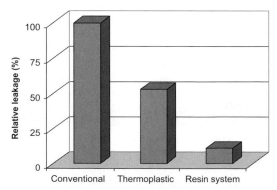

Fig. 4. Relative leakage behavior of endodontic obturation techniques. (*From* Von Fraunhofer JA. Dental materials at a glance. Oxford: Wiley-Blackwell; 2009; with permission.)

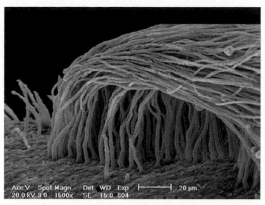

Fig. 5. FESE micrograph of EndoREZ tags extruding from the root filling material extending distances of at least 400 to 600 μm. The foreground shows fractured resin tags (caused by polymerization shrinkage) or resin tags that have partially entered the dentinal tubules. (*From* http://www.ineedce.com. Pameijer CH, Barnett F, Zmener O, Schein B. Methacrylate based resin endodontic sealers: a paradigm shift in endodontics? ENDO0710DE; 2008:1–11; with permission.)

of light from the moisture on the surface of a preparation can be visualized, in a root canal this is not possible, thus making clinical judgment more difficult.

In a study by Zmener and colleagues[14] 4 scenarios of dentin wetness or dryness were tested for apical and coronal dye leakage. In Group 1, 95% ethanol was used followed by paper points to dry the canals. In Group 2, the canals were blot dried with several paper points. In Group 3, a luer vacuum adaptor with low vacuum for 5 seconds followed by 1 paper point for only 1 to 2 seconds was used. In Group 4, the root canal remained flooded and no effort was made to remove excess distilled water. It was theorized that perhaps the hydrophilic properties of EndoREZ with the scenario in Group 4 would displace excess water.

Positive and negative controls were also tested. Dye leakage as determined by methylene blue, showed that EndoREZ and Epiphany/Resilon in Groups 2 and 3

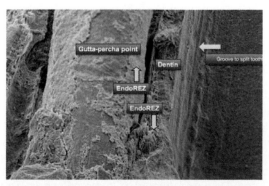

Fig. 6. Scanning electron micrograph of a gutta-percha point partially covered with EndoREZ. The space between point and adjacent dentin wall is filled with EndoREZ; however, no penetration into the dentinal tubules was observed. This is the result of over drying. (*From* Becce, C, Pameijer CH. SEM study of a new endodontic root canal sealer. J Dent Res 2001;79(AADR issue):abstract #866; with permission.)

exhibited significantly less coronal and apical leakage ($P<.05$) than Groups 1 and 4. The method with a low vacuum luer adaptor and paper point drying for 1 to 2 seconds (Group 3) scored the lowest leakage. There was no statistically significant difference between EndoREZ and Epiphany/Resilon. Another clinical technique to maintain moist dentin is to make sure that when excess water (or EDTA, saline or chlorhexidine) is removed with paper points, the last paper point shows at least 3 mm of moisture.

OXYGEN-INHIBITED LAYER

When conducting biocompatibility studies using subcutaneous implantation or intra-osseous bone implants, specimen preparation of MBRS may result in the formation of an oxygen-inhibited layer, which depends on the method of sample preparation. The presence of an oxygen-inhibited layer plays a significant role in the outcome of tissue reactions, because resin, whether chemical, light, or dual cured, does not polymerize at its surface when in contact with air. This surface layer contains unreacted monomers that are highly toxic. However, this does not mean that polymerized sealers cannot cause irritation. Conversion of monomer in a typical polymerization reaction is at best less than 70%.[52] It is important to thoroughly flush the root canal with EDTA after using NaOCl, followed by an optional final flush with sterile saline or 2% chlorhexidine (Consepsis, Ultradent Products Inc), because oxygen left behind from the NaOCl inhibits polymerization, thus forming an oxygen-inhibited layer. The effect of this was demonstrated by the following study dealing with irrigation.

IRRIGATION PROTOCOL

Bond strength values of MBRS using different intracanal irrigation scenarios vary depending on the sequence of rinses and the composition of the last rinse. To determine the importance of an irrigation protocol that does not interfere with dentin bonding of a sealer, an experiment using a modification of the thin-slice push-out test design was used by Pameijer and Zmener.[53] Intact human teeth were instrumented according to a standardized protocol and subsequently prepared to produce 18 standardized dentin tubes (n = 6 per group for 3 groups), with a 3 mm internal diameter. The irrigation protocol was as follows:

Group 1 (n = 6): irrigation for 1 minute with 10 mL of 17% EDTA to remove the smear layer followed by a continuous flow of 10 mL of 5.25% NaOCl. The canal was then dried with a luer low vacuum tip for 2 seconds followed by sterile cotton pellets leaving the dentin slightly moist with NaOCl.

Group 2 (n = 6): irrigation with a continuous flow of 10 mL of 5.25% NaOCl followed by 10 mL of 17% EDTA (1 minute each) followed by drying with a luer low vacuum tip for 2 seconds followed by sterile cotton pellets leaving the dentinal walls slightly moist with EDTA.

Group 3 (n = 6): irrigation with a continuous flow of 10 mL of 5.25% NaOCl followed by 10 mL of 17% EDTA (1 minute each) and a final 2-minute rinse with 10 mL sterile distilled water. The canals were dried with a luer low vacuum tip for 2 seconds followed by sterile paper points leaving the dentinal walls slightly moist with distilled water.

All samples were then obturated with EndoREZ as per the manufacturer' instructions and prepared for the push-out test. **Fig. 7** shows the setup of the custom-made equipment used. Data were recorded in megaPascals (**Table 1**). The results of the push-out tests revealed that all groups had measurable adhesive properties. Group 1 showed the lowest bond strength values, whereas the values for Groups 2 and 3 were much higher. Although the results in Group 3 were slightly better, no statistically significant differences were demonstrated compared with Group 2 ($P>.05$).

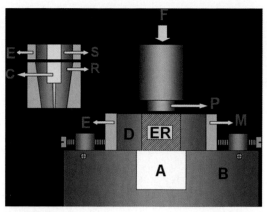

Fig. 7. The push-out test setup. A, space for displaced sealer; B, metal base of apparatus for sample fixation; F, direction of force; P, cylindrical plunger; D, 3 mm high root dentin cylinder; ER, EndoRez sealer; E and M, lateral sides of acrylic resin; R, remaining root; C, cylindrical preparation of the root canal (6 mm long with a 3 mm internal diameter); S, 3 mm high root section embedded in acrylic resin. The black line below E and S represent the cut through the samples perpendicular to the long axis of the tooth. (*From* http://www.ineedce.com. Pameijer CH, Barnett F, Zmener O, Schein B. Methacrylate based resin endodontic sealers: a paradigm shift in endodontics? ENDO0710DE; 2008:1–11; with permission.)

Visualization of the presence or absence of an oxygen-inhibited layer at the interface of dentin and EndoREZ sealer was demonstrated in cross sections (**Figs. 8** and **9**). **Fig. 8** shows a sample of Group 1. The light blue color represents dentin, the narrow gold colored band is the oxygen-inhibited layer, and the dark blue color represent fully polymerized EndoREZ. A photograph of Group 2 is significant (see **Fig. 9**) for the absence of a halo of unpolymerized resin. The dentin is light blue in color, and the dark blue represents fully polymerized EndoREZ. When EDTA was used as a final rinse, only polymerized (dark blue) EndoREZ was present at the dentin (light blue) interface and the cross sections were similar to the Group 2 samples.

It is obvious that unpolymerized resin at the interface dentin and sealer offers a pathway for leakage and has to be prevented at all cost.

CLINICAL EVIDENCE

More reports of reasonably long-term clinical studies have appeared in the literature that make it easier for the practitioner to evaluate the benefits and success of MBRS. EndoREZ was first reported on by Zmener and Pameijer.[54,55] One intermediate clinical study on Epiphany/Resilon[56] followed by a long-term clinical study have been published by Barnett and Debelian.[57]

Table 1			
Mean push-out bond strength value			
Group	n	Mean Bond Strength, MPa (SD)	Range
1	6	1.33 (0.45)	0.69–1.73
2	6	7.95 (0.60)	8.67–7.11
3	6	8.09 (0.49)	8.67–7.28

Fig. 8. Group 1 showing a cross section of dentin (*light blue*), an oxygen-inhibited layer (*gold colored halo*) and polymerized EndoREZ (*dark blue*).

In a retrospective study on 180 patients a total of 295 root canals were treated with laterally condensed gutta-percha cones in conjunction with EndoREZ. Root canal therapy was performed in 1 visit using standardized techniques. The results were assessed clinically and radiographically 14 to 24 months postoperatively[54] and after 5 years.[55] A comparison with baseline radiographs was made. Parameters for success were based on the absence of clinical symptoms, a normal or slightly widened peri-odontal ligament, and resolution of periapical radiolucencies with an absence of pain in patients who had pre-existing lesions associated with pain. After 2 years the overall success rate was 91.03%. In the subsequent 5-year follow-up that examined the same pool of patients, 129 responded to a recall request. Root canals had been adequately filled to the working length in 92 teeth (76.66%) and short in 13 (10.83%). Fifteen cases (12.50%), filled flush at the initiation of the experiment, showed slight resorption of the filling material at the apex within the lumen of the root canal. Of the 10 roots with extrusion, none had radiographic evidence of sealer in the periradicular tissues after 5 years. All patients were free of clinical symptoms. A life table analysis revealed a cumulative probability of success of 86.3% at the 5-

Fig. 9. A cross section of dentin (*light blue*), adjacent to fully polymerized ER (*dark blue*). No oxygen-inhibited layer is present.

year recall with a 95% confidence interval of 79.7 to 91.0. This percentage compares favorably with the literature[34,58,59] on the use of conventional sealers.

An example from the 5-year study is shown in the following 3 radiographs. Preoperative (**Fig. 10**A) and immediate postoperative view (**Fig. 10**B), and a 5-year follow-up (**Fig. 10**C) on tooth number 8 filled with EndoREZ and gutta-percha. Extruded sealer was resorbed during the interim and new bone was deposited. The patient has been free of symptoms since completion of treatment.

The results of Resilon/Epiphany in a 2-year prospective study have been reported by Debelian.[56] A total of 67 vital teeth were treated in 1 visit and 53 necrotic pulps in 2 visits (n = 120). After 2 years 108 cases were evaluated by 3 evaluators and the mean of the Periapical Index Scores (PAI) was calculated. When PAI 1 and 2 were combined (PAI 1 = healed; PAI 2 = in the process of healing), the success rate after 24 months was 91.6% (a similar success rate, ie, 91.3%, was reported by Zmener and Pameijer).[54]

Results after 4 years:
   86 of 102 teeth (93.1%) were scored as successful (PAI 1, 2). 53 of 56 teeth (94.6%) that were without preoperative apical periodontitis were scored as successful.
   42 of 46 teeth (91.3%) that were diagnosed as nonvital pulps with apical periodontitis were scored as successful.

Comparison between EndoREZ and Resilon is not feasible here because of the difference in evaluation periods (4 and 5 years, respectively). However, the

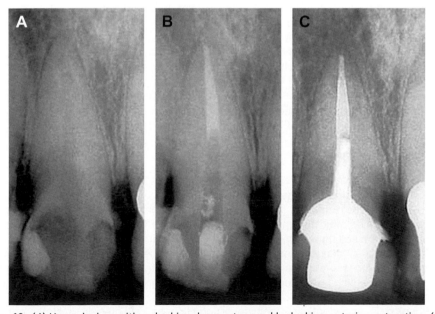

Fig. 10. (A) Upper incisor with pulpal involvement caused by leaking anterior restoration. (B) Immediate postoperative view. (C) After 5 years, the incisor, restored with a post and core and porcelain fused to metal is functional and completely asymptomatic. (From http://www. ineedce.com. Pameijer CH, Barnett F, Zmener O, Schein B. Methacrylate based resin endodontic sealers: a paradigm shift in endodontics? ENDO0710DE; 2008:1–11; with permission.)

percentages seem to indicate that both perform equally well and compare favorably with conventional sealers that have been reported in the literature.[60–62]

Ideally, more prospective clinical studies are needed to confirm these studies.

DO RESIN-BASED SEALERS REINFORCE ROOTS?

Intraradicular dentin bond strength tests have been conducted by means of a push-out test evaluating various sealers and combinations of sealers and points.

Some investigators reported higher values with resin-based sealers,[63,64] whereas others reported a lack of reinforcement.[65,66] Furthermore some experimental designs are suspect because of the drying of the root canal technique that has been discussed previously or the lack of standardization of the samples. Optimum standardization by Grande and colleagues[66] led to the following conclusion: the currently available endodontic filling materials and their recommended adhesive procedures are not able to influence the mechanical properties of root canal dentin. The flexural properties of Resilon and gutta-percha or EndoREZ and gutta-percha are too low to reinforce roots.

RETREATMENT OF MBRS

One of the requirements of a root canal sealer is that, in case of failure, the root canals can be retreated. According to de Oliveira and colleagues[67] and Ezzie and colleagues,[68] Epiphany/Resilon could be removed faster and with less residual filling material when K3 files,[67] or ProFile 0.06 combined with heat and chloroform[68] were used compared with gutta-percha and AH Plus. Automated[69] instrumentation can also be used to remove resin-based, zinc oxide, and eugenol endodontic sealers when retreating root canals. Straight canals obturated with gutta-percha and sealer may be negotiated with engine-driven stainless steel Anatomic Endodontic Technology (Ultradent Products Inc) instruments. The flute design with sharp cutting edges resulted in efficient cutting of the gutta-percha, aided by the softening of the material caused by frictional heat. Each individual instrument was discarded after instrumentation of 2 teeth, thus reducing the possibility of instrument breakage. The recommendation to use new instruments had been reported previously.[70] However, only teeth with straight canals were tested and consequently no conclusions can be drawn about the retreatment efficacy of AET instruments in curved root canals.

FUTURE EXPECTATIONS

It is anticipated that the MBRS will continue to appeal to the dental profession. New techniques and modifications of existing ones will be developed and introduced. For instance, the EndoREZ system recommends harpooning of catalyst-coated accessory cones after placement of the master cone into the sealer. This not only accelerates the setting reaction but also reduces the amount of sealer, thus reducing polymerization shrinkage; consequently a reduction in leakage can be accomplished. Because the accessory cones are placed after the master cone has been seated, there is no risk of pressing unreacted catalyst beyond the apex potentially causing damage to the periradicular tissues.

Bonding in endodontics is gaining recognition as reflected in a statement by Mounce[71]: "Given the long-term trends in dentistry there can be little, if any, doubt that the future of endodontics is bonded. The goal of being able to bond a canal from the minor constriction to the canal orifice to the occlusal surface is a desirable one."

On the challenging side of the positive ex vivo and in vivo studies and clinical success are publications that underscore the complexity of chemical compositions and their biologic interaction of currently available dental materials; these publications cannot be ignored. Material composition seems to be a critical factor.[72,73] It has been established that the co-monomer triethylene glycol dimethacrylate (TEGDMA) causes gene mutations in vitro. Formation of micronuclei indicates chromosomal damage and the induction of DNA strand breaks detected with monomers, such as TEGDMA and HEMA. New findings indicate that increased oxidative stress results in impairment of the cellular pro- and antioxidant redox balance caused by monomers. Monomers reduce the levels of the natural radical scavenger glutathione (GSH), which protects cell structures from damage caused by reactive oxygen species (ROS). Depletion of the intracellular GSH pool may then significantly contribute to cytotoxicity, because a related increase in ROS levels can activate pathways leading to apoptosis. Neither EndoREZ nor Epiphany contain these components.

After a thorough review of the available data and despite the contradicting ex vivo and in vivo tests, it seems that MBRS are here to stay. EndoREZ and Resilon are now being used successfully, about 10 years after their inception. The only conclusive evidence is long-term clinical success. Therefore more long-term data are needed to determine whether they will eventually replace conventional sealers or will be used in parallel as an alternative choice when filling root canals.

REFERENCES

1. Buonocore MG. A simple method of increasing the adhesion of acrylic filling materials to enamel surfaces. J Dent Res 1955;34:849–53.
2. Tidmarsh BG. Acid-cleaned and resin sealed root canals. J Endod 1978;4:117–21.
3. Osorio R, Erhardt MC, Pimenta LA, et al. EDTA treatment improves resin-dentin bonds' resistance to degradation. J Dent Res 2005;84:736–40.
4. Yamada R, Armas A, Goldman M, et al. A scanning electron microscopic comparison of a high volume final flush with several irrigating solutions. Part 3. J Endod 1983;9:137–42.
5. Baumgartner JC, Mader CL. A scanning electron microscopic evaluation of four root canal irrigation regimens. J Endod 1987;13:147–57.
6. Zidan O, El Deeb ME. The use of a dentinal bonding agent as a root canal sealer. J Endod 1985;11:176–8.
7. Leonard JE, Gutmann JI, Guo IY. Apical and coronal seal of roots obturated with a dentine bonding agent and resin. Int Endod J 1996;29:76–83.
8. Nikaido T, Takano Y, Sasafuchi Y, et al. Bond strengths to endodontically treated teeth. Am J Dent 1999;12:177–80.
9. Morris MD, Lee KW, Agee KA, et al. Effects of sodium hypochlorite and RC-Prep on bond strengths of resin cement to endodontic surfaces. J Endod 2001;27:753–7.
10. Erdemir A, Eldeniz AU, Belli S, et al. Effect of solvents on bonding to root canal dentin. J Endod 2004;30:589–92.
11. Manocci F, Ferrari M. Apical seal of roots obturated with laterally condensed gutta-percha, epoxy resin cement and dentin bonding agent. J Endod 1998;24:41–4.
12. Ahlberg KM, Tay WM. A methacrylate-based cement used as a root canal sealer. Int Endod J 1998;31:15–21.

13. Kataoka H, Yoshioka T, Suda H, et al. Dentin bonding and sealing ability of a new root canal resin sealer. J Endod 2000;26:230–5.
14. Zmener O, Pameijer CH, Serrano SA, et al. The significance of moist root canal dentin with the use of methacrylate-based endodontic sealers: an in vitro coronal dye leakage study. J Endod 2008;34:76–9.
15. Wong Y, Spencer P. Continuity etching of an all-in-one adhesive in wet dentin tubules. J Dent Res 2005;84:350–4.
16. Zmener O, Pameijer CH. Resin-coated gutta-percha cones coupled with a resin-based sealer: a new alternative for filling root canals. Endod Prac 2007;10:21–5.
17. Tay FR, Hiraishi N, Pashley DH, et al. Bondability of Resilon to a methacrylate-based root canal sealer. J Endod 2006;32:133–7.
18. Louw NP, Pameijer CH, Norval G. Histopathological evaluation of root canal sealer in subhuman primates. J Dent Res 2001;80(Special issue):654 [abstract #1019].
19. Becce C, Pameijer CH. SEM study of a new endodontic root canal sealer. J Dent Res 2001;79(AADR issue) [abstract #866].
20. Becce C, Pameijer CH. Biocompatibility of a new endodontic sealer. J Dent Res 2003;81(IADR Special issue):B321 [abstract #2483].
21. Huang TH, Lee H, Kao CT. Evaluation of the genotoxicity of zinc oxide eugenol-based, calcium hydroxide-based, and epoxy resin-based root canal sealers by comet assay. J Endod 2001;27:744–8.
22. Huang FM, Tai KW, Chou MY, et al. Cytotoxicity of resin-, zinc oxide-eugenol-, and calcium hydroxide-based root canal sealers on human periodontal ligament cells and permanent V79 cells. Int Endod J 2002;35:153–8.
23. Koulaouzidou EA, Papazisis KT, Beltes P, et al. Cytotoxicity of three resin-based root canal sealers: an in vitro evaluation. Endod Dent Traumatol 1998;14:182–5.
24. Bouillaguet S, Wataha JC, Tay FR, et al. Initial in vitro biological response to contemporary endodontic sealers. J Endod 2006;32:989–92.
25. Key JE, Rahemtulla FG, Eleazer PD. Cytotoxicity of a new root canal filling material on human gingival fibroblasts. J Endod 2006;32:756–8.
26. Eldeniz AU, Mustafa K, Ørstavik D, et al. Cytotoxicity of new resin-, calcium hydroxide-and silicone-based root canal sealers on fibroblasts derived from human gingiva and L929 cell lines. Int Endod J 2007;40:329–37.
27. Lodiene G, Morisbak E, Bruzell E, et al. Toxicity evaluation of root canal sealers in vitro. Int Endod J 2008;41:72–7.
28. Oliver CM, Abbott PV. Correlation between clinical success and apical dye penetration. Int Endod J 2001;34:637–44.
29. Zmener O. Tissue response to a new methacrylate-based root canal sealer: preliminary observations in the subcutaneous connective tissue of rats. J Endod 2004;30:348–51.
30. Zmener O, Pameijer CH, Banegas G. Bone tissue response to a methacrylate-based endodontic sealer: a histological and histometric study. J Endod 2005; 31:457–9.
31. Sousa CJ, Montes CR, Pascon EA, et al. Comparison of the intraosseous biocompatibility of AH Plus, EndoREZ, and Epiphany root canal sealers. J Endod 2006; 32:656–62.
32. Ferracane JL, Condon JR. Rate of elution of leachable components from composite. Dent Mater 1990;6:282–7.
33. Spångberg LS. In vitro assessment of the toxicity of endodontic materials. Int Endod J 1981;14:27–34.
34. Orstavik D, Kerekes K, Eriksen HM. Clinical performance of three endodontic sealers. Endod Dent Traumatol 1987;3:178–86.

35. Zmener O, Banegas G. Apical leakage of endodontic sealers. Endod Pract 2004; 7:30–2.
36. Orucoglu H, Sengun A, Yilmaz N. Apical leakage of resin based root canal sealers with a new computerized fluid filtration meter. J Endod 2005;31:886–90.
37. Da Silva Neto UX, de Moraes IG, Westphalen VP, et al. Leakage of 4 resin-based root-canal sealers used with a single-cone technique. Oral Surg Oral Med Oral Pathol Oral Radiol Endod 2007;104:e53–7.
38. Adanir N, Cobankara FK, Belli S. Sealing properties of different resin-based root canal sealers. J Biomed Mater Res B Appl Biomater 2006;77:1–4.
39. Onay EO, Ungor M, Orucoglu H. An in vitro evaluation of the apical sealing ability of a new resin-based root canal obturation system. J Endod 2006;32:976–8.
40. Tunga U, Bodrumlu E. Assessment of the sealing ability of a new root canal obturation material. J Endod 2006;32:876–8.
41. Stratton RK, Apicella MJ, Mines P. A fluid filtration comparison of gutta-percha versus Resilon, a new soft resin endodontic obturation system. J Endod 2006; 32:642–5.
42. Shipper G, Orstavik D, Teixeira FB, et al. An evaluation of microbial leakage in roots filled with a thermoplastic synthetic polymer-based root canal filling material (Resilon). J Endod 2004;30:342–7.
43. Maltezos C, Glickman GN, Ezzo P, et al. Comparison of the sealing of Resilon, Pro Root MTA, and Super-EBA as root-end filling materials: a bacterial leakage study. J Endod 2006;32:324–7.
44. Pitout E, Oberholzer TG, Blignaut E, et al. Coronal leakage of teeth root-filled with gutta-percha or Resilon root canal filling material. J Endod 2006;32:879–81.
45. Biggs SG, Knowles KI, Ibarrola JL, et al. An in vitro assessment of the sealing ability of Resilon/Epiphany using fluid filtration. J Endod 2006;32:759–61.
46. Gernhardt CR, Kruger T, Bekes K, et al. Apical sealing ability of 2 epoxy resin-based sealers used with root canal obturation techniques based on warm gutta-percha compared to cold lateral condensation. Quintessence Int 2007;38:229–34.
47. Sevimay S, Kalayci A. Evaluation of apical sealing ability and adaptation to dentine of two resin-based sealers. J Oral Rehabil 2005;32:105–10.
48. Aptekar A, Ginnan K. Comparative analysis of microleakage and seal for 2 obturation materials: Resilon/Epiphany and gutta-percha. J Can Dent Assoc 2006;72:245.
49. Wu MK, Wesselink PR. Endodontic leakage studies reconsidered. Part I. Methodology, application, and relevance. Int Endod J 1993;26:37–43.
50. von Fraunhofer JA, Kurtzman GM, Norby CE. Resin-based sealing of root canals in endodontic therapy. Gen Dent 2006;54:243–6.
51. Kardon BP, Kuttler S, Hardigan P, et al. An in vitro evaluation of the sealing ability of a new root-canal-obturation system. J Endod 2003;29:658–61.
52. Kidal KK, Ruyter IE. How different curing methods affect the degree of conversion of resin-based inlay/onlay materials. Acta Odontol Scand 1994;52:315–22.
53. Pameijer CH, Zmener O. The effect of irrigation protocol on the polymerization of resin-based sealers–significance of oxygen inhibition. In: Methacrylate based resin sealers – a paradigm shift in endodontics. South Jordan (UT): Ultradent Press; 2009. p. 135.
54. Zmener O, Pameijer CH. Clinical and radiographic evaluation of a resin-based root canal sealer. Am J Dent 2004;17:19–22.
55. Zmener O, Pameijer CH. Clinical and radiographical evaluation of a resin-based root canal sealer: a 5-year follow-up. J Endod 2007;33:676–9.
56. Debelian G. Treatment outcome of teeth treated with an evidenced-based disinfection protocol and filled with Resilon. J Endod 2006;32 [abstract #PR4].

57. Barnett F, Debelian G. Clinical outcomes of endodontically treated teeth filled with Resilon. In: Methacrylate based resin sealers–a paradigm shift in endodontics. South Jordan (UT): Ultradent Press; 2009. p. 119.
58. Friedman S, Löst C, Zarrabian M, et al. Evaluation of success and failure after endodontic therapy using a glass ionomer cement sealer. J Endod 1995;21:384–90.
59. Huumonen S, Lenander-Lumikari M, Sigurdsson A, et al. Healing of apical periodontitis after endodontic treatment: a comparison between a silicone-based and a zinc oxide-eugenol-based sealer. Int Endod J 2003;36:296–301.
60. Kerekes K, Tronstad L. Long-term results of endodontic treatment performed with a standardized technique. J Endod 1979;5:83–90.
61. Hoskinson SE, Ng YL, Hoskinson AE, et al. A retrospective comparison of outcome of root canal treatment using two different protocols. Oral Surg Oral Med Oral Pathol Oral Radiol Endod 2002;93:705–15.
62. Field JW, Gutmann JL, Solomon ES, et al. A clinical radiographic retrospective assessment of the success rate of single-visit root canal treatment. Int Endod J 2004;37:70–82.
63. Skidmore LJ, Berzins DW, Bahcall JK. An in vitro comparison of the inraradicular dentin bond strength of Resilon and gutta-percha. J Endod 2006;32:963–6.
64. Teixeira FB, Teixeira EC, Thompson JY, et al. Fracture resistance of roots endodontically treated with a new resin filling material. J Am Dent Assoc 2004;135:646–52.
65. Ungor M, Onay EO, Orucoglu H. Push-out bond strengths: the Epiphany-Resilon endodontic obturation system compared with different pairings of Epiphany, Resilon, AH Plus and gutta-percha. Int Endod J 2006;39:643–7.
66. Grande NM, Lavorgna L, Ioppolo P, et al. Influence of different root canal filling materials on the mechanical properties of root canal dentin. J Endod 2007;33:859–64.
67. de Oliveira DP, Barbizam JV, Trope M, et al. Comparison between gutta-percha and resilon removal using two different techniques in endodontic retreatment. J Endod 2006;32:362–4.
68. Ezzie E, Fleury A, Solomon E, et al. Efficacy of retreatment techniques for a resin-based root canal obturation material. J Endod 2006;32:341–4.
69. Zmener O, Banegas G, Pameijer CH. Efficacy of an automated instrumentation technique in removing resin-based and zinc oxide and eugenol endodontic sealers when retreating root canals: An in vitro study. Endod Prac 2005;8:29–33.
70. Tronstad L, Niemczyk SP. Efficacy and safety tests of six automated devices for root canal instrumentation. Endod Dent Traumatol 1986;2:270–6.
71. Mounce R. Say what you will: the future of endodontic obturation is bonded. Endod Prac 2007;10:48.
72. Schweikl H, Spagnuolo G, Schmalz G. Genetic and cellular toxicology of dental resin monomers. J Dent Res 2006;85:870–7.
73. Schweikl H, Hartmann A, Hiller KA, et al. Inhibition of TEGDMA and HEMA-induced genotoxicity and cell cycle arrest by N-acetylcysteine. Dent Mater 2007;23:688–95.

The Endo-Restorative Interface: Current Concepts

Marga Ree, DDS, MSc[a], Richard S. Schwartz, DDS[b,c],*

KEYWORDS
- Endodontics • Restorative dentistry
- Adhesive dentistry • Posts

The primary goals of endodontic treatment are straightforward: to debride and disinfect the root canal space to the greatest possible extent, and then seal the canals as effectively as possible. The materials and techniques change somewhat over time, but not the ultimate goals. The primary goals of restorative treatment are to restore teeth to function and comfort and in some cases, aesthetics. Once again, the materials and techniques change, but not the ultimate goals of treatment. Successful endodontic treatment depends on the restorative treatment that follows. The connection between endodontic treatment and restorative dentistry is well accepted, but the best restorative approaches for endodontically treated teeth have always been somewhat controversial. The topic is no less controversial today, despite the massive (and ever growing) amount of information available from research, journal articles, courses, "expert" opinions, and various sources from the Internet. In fact, information overload contributes to the controversy because so much of it is contradictory.

With the emergence of implants into the mainstream of dentistry, there has been more emphasis on long-term outcomes and on evaluating the "restorability" of teeth prior to endodontic treatment. Patients are not well served if the endodontic treatment is successful but the tooth fails. The long-term viability of endodontically treated teeth is no longer a "given" in the implant era. In consequence, some teeth that might have received endodontic treatment in the past are now extracted and replaced with implant-supported prostheses if they are marginally restorable or it makes more sense in the overall treatment plan. It is not possible to review in one article all the literature on the restoration of endodontically treated teeth. This article therefore focuses primarily on current concepts based on the literature from the past 10 years or so, and provides treatment guidelines based on that research.

[a] Meeuwstraat 110, 1444 VH Purmerend, Netherlands
[b] 1130 East Sonterra Boulevard, Suite 140, San Antonio, TX 78258, USA
[c] University of Texas Health Science Center at San Antonio, San Antonio, TX, USA
* Corresponding author. 1130 East Sonterra Boulevard, Suite 140, San Antonio, TX 78258.
E-mail address: sasunny@satx.rr.com

Dent Clin N Am 54 (2010) 345–374
doi:10.1016/j.cden.2009.12.005
0011-8532/10/$ – see front matter © 2010 Elsevier Inc. All rights reserved.

THE RELATIONSHIP BETWEEN ENDODONTICS AND RESTORATIVE DENTISTRY

Long-term success of endodontic treatment is highly dependent on the restorative treatment that follows. Once restored, the tooth must be structurally sound and the disinfected status of the root canal system must be maintained. Because microorganisms are known to be the primary etiologic factor for apical periodontitis[1] and endodontic failure,[2] contamination of the root canal system during or after restorative treatment is considered an important factor in the ultimate success or failure. Exposure of gutta-percha to saliva in the pulp chamber results in migration of bacteria to the apex in a matter of days.[3] Endotoxin reaches the apex even faster.[4] The importance of the coronal restoration in successful endodontic treatment has been shown in several studies.[5,6] Delayed restoration has been show to result in lower success rates.[7]

Successful restorative treatment is also greatly influenced by the execution of the endodontic procedures. Radicular and coronal tooth structure should be preserved to the greatest possible extent during endodontic procedures.[8–10] Root canal preparations should attempt to preserve dentin in the coronal one-third of the root. There is no reason to prepare a "coke bottle" type of canal preparation (**Fig. 1**) that weakens the tooth unnecessarily. Access preparations similarly should be made in such a way that cervical dentin is preserved. The roof of the pulp chamber should be removed carefully, preserving the walls of the chamber as much as possible. The chamber walls should be prepared only to the extent that is necessary for adequate access for endodontic treatment.

Many, if not most endodontically treated teeth today are restored with adhesive materials. Adhesive materials provide an immediate seal and some immediate strengthening of the tooth. These materials are generally not dependent on gross mechanical retention, so tooth structure can be preserved. The sections that follow discuss basic principles of adhesive dentistry and some of the limitations, pitfalls, and special problems presented by endodontically treated teeth.

BONDING TO ENAMEL

Enamel is a highly mineralized tissue that is often present along the margins of access preparations of anterior teeth and sometimes in posterior teeth. Effective bonding

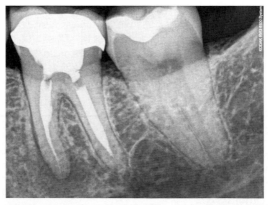

Fig. 1. This radiograph shows canals prepared with a "coke bottle" design. Excessive dentin was removed in the cervical one-third of the root and the apical preparations are thin.

procedures for enamel were first reported in 1955.[11] An acid, such as 30% to 40% phosphoric acid, when applied to enamel will cause selective dissolution of the enamel prisms. Microporosities are created within and around the enamel prisms, which can be infiltrated with a low-viscosity resin and polymerized,[12] creating resin "tags" that provide micromechanical retention and a strong, durable bond. It is important to prevent contamination of etched enamel with blood, saliva, or moisture that will interfere with bonding.[13] Poorly etched enamel leads to staining at the margins of the restoration.[14] A good enamel bond protects the less durable underlying dentin bond.[15]

BONDING TO METAL-CERAMIC AND ALL-CERAMIC RESTORATIONS

Access cavities are often made through metal-ceramic or all-ceramic materials, so attaining an effective, durable bond is important. Like enamel, the porcelain margins can be etched (usually with a 1-minute etch of 10% hydrofluoric acid) to create microporosities, which may be infiltrated with resin and polymerized. Application of silane to the etched porcelain surface enhances the bond.[16] Etched ceramic materials form a strong, durable bond with resin.[17]

BONDING TO DENTIN: RESIN-BASED MATERIALS

A smear layer is formed when the dentin surface is cut or abraded with hand or rotary instruments. The smear layer adheres to the dentin surface and plugs the dentinal tubules; it consists of ground-up collagen and hydroxyapatite and other substances that might be present such as bacteria, salivary components, or pulpal remnants.[18] The smear layer cannot be rinsed or rubbed off,[19] but can be removed with an acid or chelating agent. Some dentin adhesives remove the smear layer, whereas others penetrate through the layer and incorporate it into the bond. Both approaches may be used successfully.[12]

Bonding to dentin is more complex than bonding to enamel or ceramic. Dentin is a wet substrate and restorative resins are hydrophobic ("water hating"). Dentin consists of approximately 50% inorganic mineral (hydroxyapatite) by volume, 30% organic components (primarily type 1 collagen), and 20% fluid.[20] The wet environment and relative lack of a mineralized surface made the development of effective dentin adhesives a challenge.

The first successful strategy for dentin adhesion was reported by Nakabayashi and colleagues in 1982.[21] Their ideas were not widely accepted until later in the decade. Nakabayashi showed that resin could be bonded to dentin by demineralizing the dentin surface and applying an intermediate layer that would bond to dentin and restorative materials. Although not as durable and reliable as enamel bonding, dentin bonding forms the foundation for many of today's restorative procedures. Nakabayashi's technique was later simplified by combining some of the steps.

THE LIMITATIONS OF DENTIN BONDING

From the restorative literature it is known that dentin bonding materials have limitations, many of which are related to polymerization shrinkage. When resin-based materials polymerize, individual monomer molecules join to form chains that contract as the chains grow and intertwine, and the mass undergoes volumetric shrinkage.[22] Resin-based restorative materials shrink from 2% to 7%, depending on the volume occupied by filler particles and the test method.[23-25] The force of polymerization contraction often exceeds the bond strength of dentin adhesives to dentin, resulting in gap formation along the surfaces with the weakest bonds.[26] Resins, even in thin layers, generate very high forces from polymerization contraction.[27,28]

Another limitation of dentin bonding is deterioration of the resin bond over time. This process is well documented in vitro[15,29–31] and in vivo.[32,33] Loss of bond strength is first detectable in the laboratory at 3 months.[30] Interfacial leakage increases as the bond degrades.[22,34] Functional forces have been shown to contribute to the degradation of the resin bond in restorative applications.[30,35]

THE LIMITATIONS OF BONDING IN THE ROOT CANAL SYSTEM

The root canal system has an unfavorable geometry for resin bonding.[36] Configuration factor or C-Factor, the ratio of bonded to unbonded resin surfaces,[23] is often used as a quantitative measure of the geometry of the cavity preparation for bonding. The greater the percentage of unbonded surfaces, the less stress is placed on the bonded surfaces from polymerization contraction. The unbonded surfaces allow plastic deformation or flow within the resin mass during polymerization.[23,37] A Class 4 cavity preparation, for example, has a favorable geometry with a ratio of less than 1:1. There are few if any walls that directly oppose each other, and more than half of the resin surfaces are not bonded. In the root canal system the ratio might be 100:1,[23] because virtually every dentin wall has an opposing wall and there are minimal unbonded surfaces. Any ratio greater than 3:1 is considered unfavorable for bonding.[38] Because of this unfavorable geometry, it is not possible to achieve the gap-free interface with current materials. Interfacial gaps are virtually always present in bonded restorations in restorative dentistry,[39] obturating materials,[40] and bonded posts,[41,42] and gap formation increases with time.[43]

THE POTENTIAL PROBLEMS OF USING ADHESIVE MATERIALS DEEP IN THE ROOT CANAL SYSTEM

Performing the bonding steps is problematic deep in the root canal system. Uniform application of a primer or adhesive can be difficult. Once the primer is applied, the volatile carrier must be evaporated. This process can also be problematic deep in the canal. If the acetone or alcohol carrier is not completely removed, the bond is adversely affected.[44] An in vitro post study by Bouillaguet and colleagues[45] reported lower bond strengths were achieved bonding in the root canal system than bonding to flat prepared samples of radicular dentin.

COMPATIBILITY PROBLEMS WITH DUAL-CURE AND SELF-CURE RESINS

Because penetration with a curing light is limited in the root canal system, dual-cure or self-cure resin adhesives must be used. Dual-cure resins contain components that provide rapid light polymerization in those areas where the curing light penetrates effectively and a slower chemical polymerization in those areas where the light is not effective. Adhesives and sealers that contain a self-cure component have compatibility problems with self-etching dentin adhesive systems (ie, sixth and seventh generation), so they should be used with "fourth generation" etch-and-rinse adhesives.[41,46,47]

IRRIGATING SOLUTIONS AND MEDICAMENTS

Sodium hypochlorite is commonly used as an endodontic irrigant because of its antimicrobial and tissue dissolving properties. The antimicrobial properties of sodium hypochlorite are largely due to it being a strong oxidizing agent, but as a result it leaves behind an oxygen-rich layer on the dentin surface. The same applies to chelating agents that contain hydrogen peroxide. Oxygen is one of the many substances that inhibit the polymerization of resins. When dentin bonding agents are applied to an oxygen-rich surface, low bond strengths are achieved[48–50] and microleakage is increased.[51] A reducing agent, such as ascorbic acid and sodium ascorbate, applied to the dentin surface will reverse the negative affects of sodium hypochlorite.[48,51] A final soak with ethylenediamine tetra-acetic acid (EDTA) has also been reported to be effective.[52]

BASIC PRINCIPLES FOR RESTORING ENDODONTICALLY TREATED TEETH

Although many aspects of the restoration of endodontically treated remain controversial, there are several areas of general agreement. One of the best documented principles is cuspal coverage. Several studies evaluated factors that affected the survival of endodontically treated teeth. Cuspal coverage was the most consistent finding.[53–55] In one study, teeth with cuspal coverage had a 6 times greater survival rate than teeth without cuspal coverage.[56] Another study showed teeth without cuspal coverage had only a 36% survival rate after 5 years.[57]

Another important principle is preservation of tooth structure. Coronal tooth structure should be preserved to support the core buildup.[9,10] Several studies identify remaining coronal tooth structure as the most important factor in tooth survival in teeth with posts.[8,9,58]

As stated previously, radicular tooth structure should also be preserved. For most teeth that are to receive posts, no additional dentin should be removed beyond what is necessary to complete the endodontic treatment. If a tooth is prepared for a 0.06 tapered preparation, a 0.06 tapered post should "drop right in" without removing additional radicular dentin.

There is wide general agreement that the "ferrule effect" is important. In dentistry, the ferrule refers to the cervical tooth structure that provides retention and resistance form to the restoration and protects it from fracture. In one study, teeth with a ferrule of 1 mm of vertical tooth structure doubled the resistance to fracture compared with teeth restored without a ferrule.[59] Other studies have shown maximum beneficial effects from a ferrule of 1.5 to 2 mm.[60–62] The "ferrule effect" is important to long-term success when a post is used.[61] In anterior teeth, the lingual aspect of the ferrule is the most important part.[63] If the height of the remaining dentin is not sufficient to create an adequate ferrule, crown lengthening, orthodontic extrusion, or extraction may be indicated.

TEETH RESTORED WITH POSTS

Endodontically treated teeth often have substantial loss of tooth structure and require a core buildup. If retention and resistance of the core are compromised, a post may also be necessary. Custom cast posts and cores or prefabricated metal posts were the standard for many years. In the past 10 years or so, fiber-reinforced composite posts have gained popularity.

INDICATIONS FOR A POST

The primary function of a post is to retain a core in a tooth with extensive loss of coronal tooth structure.[64] Posts should not be placed arbitrarily, however, because preparation of a post channel adds a degree of risk to a restorative procedure:

- Disturbing the seal of the root canal filling, which may lead to microleakage[65,66]

- Removal of sound tooth structure, which weakens the root and may result in premature loss due to root fracture[67,68]
- Increased risk of perforation.[69]

Some studies report higher failure rates in endodontically treated teeth with posts than without.[7,70] The finding was not universal, however.[71]

Traditional thought has been that posts do not "reinforce" the root; this was apparently true for metal posts,[72,73] but there is a growing body of evidence that fiber posts may strengthen the root and make it more resistant to fracture. To date, 9 studies have shown a strengthening effect[74–82] while 3 have shown no effect.[10,83,84]

Metal posts have a high modulus of elasticity, which means that they are stiff and able to withstand forces without distortion. When a force is placed on a tooth containing a stiff post, it is transmitted to the less rigid root dentin, and concentrates at the apex of the post. Stress concentration in the post/root complex increases the chances of fracture.

To overcome the concerns about unfavorable stress distribution generated by metal posts, fiber-reinforced composite resin posts were introduced in 1990, with the aim of providing more elastic support to the core. The reduced stress transfer to tooth structure was claimed to reduce the likelihood of root fracture.[85] Posts made of materials with a modulus of elasticity similar to dentin are more resilient, absorb more impact force, and distribute the forces better than stiffer posts.[36]

TYPES OF POSTS

Posts can be categorized by modulus of elasticity, composition, fabrication process, shape, and surface texture.

Rigid Post Systems

- Metal
  - custom cast
  - prefabricated
- Zirconium and ceramic.

Posts traditionally were made of metal, and were either custom cast or prefabricated. Custom cast posts and cores are made of precious or nonprecious casting alloys; prefabricated posts are typically made of stainless steel, nickel chromium alloy, or titanium alloy. With the exception of the titanium alloys, they are very strong.

Parallel metal posts are more retentive than tapered posts[86] and induce less stress into the root, because they have less wedging effect and are reported to be less likely to cause root fractures than tapered posts.[59,87] In a retrospective study, Sorensen and Martinoff[53] reported a higher success rate with parallel metal posts than tapered posts. Tapered posts, on the other hand, require less dentin removal because most roots are tapered.

Prefabricated posts can be further divided in active or passive posts. Most active posts are threaded and intended to engage the walls of the canal, whereas passive posts are retained primarily by the frictional retention of the luting agent. Active posts are more retentive than passive posts, but introduce more stress into the root than passive posts.[88] Active posts have very limited indications, and are only recommended when the need for retention is the overriding factor.

One factor that has reduced the use of metal posts is aesthetics. Metal posts may be visible through translucent all-ceramic restorations, and even with less translucent restorations may cause the marginal gingiva to appear dark. These concerns have led to the development of posts that are white or translucent. Among the materials used for "aesthetic" posts are zirconium and other ceramic materials. These posts will work clinically, but have several disadvantages.

Among rigid posts, zirconium is stiffer and more brittle than metal. Zirconium posts were shown to cause significantly more root fractures than fiber posts in vitro.[89,90] When compared with custom cast and fiber posts, ceramic posts had a lower failure load in vivo[91] and in vitro.[92–94] As a group, they tend to be weaker than metal posts, so a thicker post is necessary, which may require removal of additional radicular tooth structure. Zirconium posts cannot be etched, therefore it is not possible to bond a composite core material to the post, making core retention a problem.[92] Retrieval of zirconium and ceramic posts is very difficult if endodontic retreatment is necessary or if the post fractures. Some ceramic materials can be removed by grinding away the remaining post material with a bur, but this is a tedious and risky procedure. It is impossible to grind away a zirconium post. In many cases, excessive removal of dentin is necessary to remove a zirconium post. For these reasons, ceramic and zirconium posts should be avoided.

Metal and zirconium posts are all radiopaque and clearly visible on a radiograph (**Figs. 2** and **3**). The radiopacity of titanium is similar to that of gutta-percha, and therefore sometimes the presence of a titanium post is difficult to detect on radiographs (**Fig. 4**).

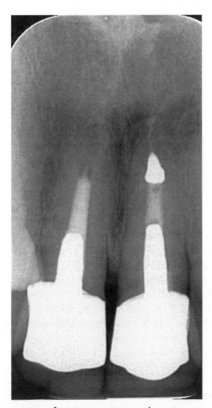

Fig. 2. Radiographic appearance of custom cast metal posts.

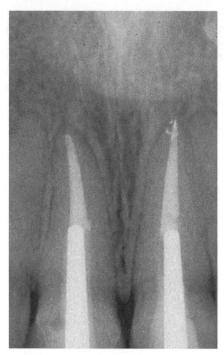

Fig. 3. Radiographic appearance of zirconium posts.

Nonrigid Post Systems: Fiber Posts

- Carbon fiber
- Glass fiber
- Quartz fiber
- Silicon fiber.

The first composite reinforced fiber posts were made with carbon fibers, which were arranged longitudinally and embedded in an epoxy resin matrix.[85] The black carbon fibers were rapidly replaced by more esthetic white and translucent glass and quartz fibers, which are now the standard components in fiber posts. These posts are commonly used in aesthetically demanding areas.

The main advantage of fiber posts is the uniform distribution of forces in the root, which results in fewer catastrophic failures than occur with metal posts if an adequate ferrule is present.[95] Several in vitro studies report that teeth restored with nonrigid posts have fewer catastrophic, irreparable root fractures when tested to failure.[96,97] Clinical studies of fiber post systems also report successful multiyear service with few or no root fractures.[8,98,99] A retrospective clinical study of carbon fiber posts and custom cast posts reported root fractures in 9% of teeth restored with cast posts, and no root fractures in teeth restored with fiber posts after 4 years.[100] In a long-term retrospective study of the clinical performance of fiber posts by Ferrari and colleagues,[8] a 7% to 11% failure rate was reported for 3 different types of fiber posts after a service period of 7 to 11 years. Half of the failures were classified as endodontic failures, the other half were mechanical failures. Out of 985 posts evaluated, the nonendodontic failures consisted of one root fracture, one fiber post fracture, 17 crown

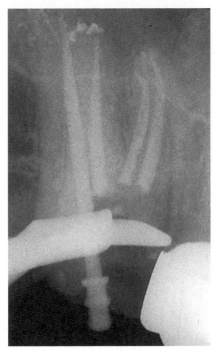

Fig. 4. Radiographic appearance of a titanium post. Note that the radiopacity of gutta-percha and titanium is very similar.

dislodgements, and 21 failures due to post debonding. The mechanical failures were always related to the lack of coronal tooth structure. In a review by Dietschi and colleagues[101] it was concluded that nonvital teeth restored with composite resin or composite resin combined with fiber posts currently represent the best treatment option.

Although fiber posts offer several advantages, they do have limitations. Posts and core foundations are subjected to repeated lateral forces in clinical function. Because nonrigid posts have a modulus of elasticity and flexural strength close to that of dentin, they flex under occlusal load. When there is an adequate ferrule, the cervical tooth structure itself resists lateral flexion.[95] However, in structurally compromised teeth that lack cervical stiffness from dentin walls and an adequate ferrule, a flexible post may result in micro-movement of the core and coronal leakage,[102,103] which in turn may lead to caries or loss of the core and crown.

Fiber posts were shown to lose flexural strength if they are submitted to cyclic loading or to thermocycling[104,105] due to degradation of the matrix in which the fibers are embedded. The strength of fiber posts varied between brands, but was directly related to post diameter and was reduced by thermocycling.[106]

Parallel fiber posts are more retentive than tapered posts.[107,108] However, in a clinical study by Signore and colleagues[99] no difference was found in the long-term survival rate of maxillary anterior teeth restored with tapered or parallel-sided glass-fiber posts and full-ceramic crown coverage. The overall survival rate was reported to be 98.5%. Most fiber posts are relatively radiolucent and have a different radiographic appearance than traditional metal posts (**Fig. 5**).

It has been shown that the retention of fiber posts relies mainly on mechanical (frictional) retention rather than bonding, similar to metal posts.[41,42,109,110] Several in vitro

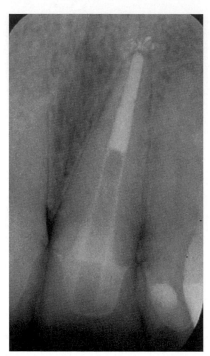

Fig. 5. Radiographic appearance of a glass-fiber post. The post is radiolucent, but the radiopaque composite clearly reveals its outline.

studies have confirmed the presence of gaps in the interface between the luting composite resin of the fiber post and the root canal wall,[42,110] and that the bond strengths between fiber posts and dentin are low, about 5 to 6 MPa.[109,111] This situation is due primarily to the unfavorable bonding environment of the root canal system, as discussed earlier.

POST LENGTH AND REMAINING ROOT CANAL FILLING

The length of a post is dictated by several factors, some of which are conflicting. Most of the studies on optimum post length were done with metal posts, but there is no compelling evidence that the principles of post length are different for fiber posts.

Braga and colleagues[112] evaluated the force required to remove glass fiber and metallic cast posts with different lengths. Irrespective the post type, posts with 10-mm length had higher retention values than posts with 6-mm length. In a study by Büttel and colleagues,[113] teeth restored with glass-fiber posts with insertion depths of 6 mm resulted in significantly higher mean failure than teeth with post space preparation of 3 mm. The retention of fiber posts was shown to be directly proportional to the insertion length in resin cubes.[114]

Several "rules" have been suggested for passively fitting posts:

- The post length below the alveolar crest should be at least equal to the length above the alveolar crest.[64,115] Sorensen and Martinoff[53] reported 97% success if post length at least equaled the crown height.
- The post should end halfway between the crestal bone and the root apex.[64]
- A post should extend at least apical to the crest of the alveolar bone.[67]

Another factor that influences post length is the length of the remaining apical root canal filling. Several studies have investigated apical seal following post space preparation and have reported that 3 to 5 mm of gutta-percha is the minimum recommended,[116–118] and longer is better[117,118]; this is sometimes dictated by the length of the canal. Post placement in a long root, for example, a canine of 28 mm, allows more apical root canal filling, as placing a 23-mm post is unnecessary. When using the criterion that the post should extend beyond the apical crest, teeth with bone loss need longer posts than teeth with normal bone height.

LIGHT-TRANSMITTING FIBER POSTS

Although it seems logical that translucent posts would transmit light for enhancement of cure deeper in the canal, there seems to be no consensus in the literature on this issue. The use of a light-transmitting translucent fiber post was reported to increase the depth of resin cure in several in vitro studies,[119–121] but other studies reported minimal or no benefits from translucent posts. One study evaluated the influence of fiber-post translucency on the degree of conversion of a dual-cure composite. Low degrees of conversion were found for the medium and deep depths.[122] Another in vitro study measured light transmission through 4 different posts of a standard length of 10 mm. All posts evaluated showed some light transmission capacity, but with values lower than 40% of incident light. One post demonstrated less than 1% light transmission.[108] Goracci and colleagues evaluated the light transmission of several fiber posts. These investigators reported no light transmission through 2 posts, and for all other posts light intensity decreased from coronal to apical, and rose again at the apical tip. Light transmission was significantly higher at the coronal level.[123] Another study showed that even without a post, the luminous intensity inside the canal decreased to levels that are insufficient for polymerization, especially in the apical third.[124] Based on these findings, the use of light-cured resin cements for post placement cannot be recommended. The benefits of light-transmitting posts are unclear.

IS THERE BENEFIT TO PLACING A POST AFTER ENDODONTIC TREATMENT OF A TOOTH WITH A CROWN?

In most cases, when preparing endodontic access through a crown there is no way of knowing the amount or strength of the underlying tooth structure, which is a particular concern in small teeth and bridge abutments.

When an access preparation is made through a crown, retention is lost.[125] When the access opening is restored with amalgam or composite resin, the retention values are restored.[125,126] When the access opening is restored with a post, the retention is greater than before the access was prepared.[125]

There is growing evidence that the insertion of a fiber post can also increase fracture resistance of teeth with crowns. An in vitro study has shown that placement of fiber posts can improve fracture resistance in maxillary premolars under full-coverage crowns.[76] The use of fiber posts in endodontically treated maxillary incisors with different types of full-coverage crowns increased their resistance to fracture[81,82] and improved the prognosis in case of fracture.[81] The type of crown was not a significant factor affecting fracture resistance, whereas the presence of a post was. D'Arcangelo and colleagues[80] showed that fiber posts significantly increased mean load values for maxillary central incisors prepared for veneers.

Based on these findings, it seems retention will be enhanced by a post, and fracture resistance will probably be improved as long as no additional tooth structure is removed. The authors routinely place fiber posts in bridge abutments and small teeth with crowns (**Fig. 6**).

POST PLACEMENT
Advantages of Immediate Post Placement

The literature on the timing of the post space preparation is inconclusive. Some studies showed less leakage after immediate post space preparation,[127,128] whereas other articles showed no difference [118,129] Some in vitro studies showed that delayed cementation of a fiber post resulted in higher retentive strengths.[130,131] Scanning electron microscopy examination revealed a more conspicuous presence of sealer remnants on the walls of immediately prepared post spaces.[131] Remnants of sealer and gutta-percha may impair adhesive bonding and resin cementation of fiber posts.[132,133] Therefore, it is important to clean the root canal walls before conditioning the dentin for post placement. Acid-etching of the prepared post space and EDTA irrigation combined with ultrasonics are reported to be an effective method.[134,135] The use of magnification can facilitate inspection of the post space for cleanliness.

Immediate preparation for post placement following obturation has several advantages. The operator has a great familiarity with the root canal morphology, working lengths, and reference points of the root canal system. In addition, placement of a temporary post and restoration can be avoided, as maintaining the temporary seal can be difficult. In vitro studies by Fox and Gutteridge[136] and by Demarchi and Sato[137] showed that teeth restored with temporary posts leaked extensively.

LUTING FIBER POSTS

Fiber posts are usually luted with lightly filled composite resins. Light penetration is limited, so dual-cure of self-cure luting resins must be used. Some luting resins are used with a separate etchant and primer (total-etch method), whereas others contain an acidic primer in the luting cement (self-etching method). More recently a third category has been added (self-adhesive method), in which there is no etching and no primer. Several studies have evaluated these luting cements.

Goracci and colleagues[138] reported that the values achieved by total-etch method were significantly higher than self-etch resin cements. Transmission electron

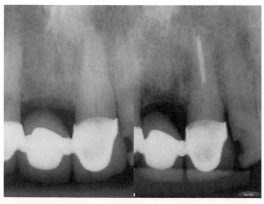

Fig. 6. The authors routinely use fiber posts when restoring access openings through crowns on bridge abutments or small teeth.

microscopy analysis revealed that the acidic resin monomers responsible for substrate conditioning in self-etch and self-adhesive resin cements did not effectively remove the thick smear layer created on root dentin during post space preparation. Valandro and colleagues[139] similarly concluded that more reliable bond strengths in the dowel space might be achieved when using total-etch adhesive systems instead of self-etching adhesives. A study by Radovic and colleagues[140] concluded that the use of self-etching resin luting systems offer less favorable adhesion to root canal dentin in comparison with the total-etch and self-adhesive approaches.

Self-adhesive cements were introduced in 2002 as a new subgroup of resin cements. Self-adhesive cements do not require any pretreatment of the tooth substrate. The cement is mixed and applied in a single clinical step. The application of self-adhesive cements to radicular dentin does not result in the formation of hybrid layer or resin tags.[138] Lührs and colleagues[141] found the shear bond strength of self-adhesive resin cements to be inferior compared with conventional composite resin cements. The sealing ability of 2 self-adhesive resin cements was shown to be significantly lower than a self-etching and 2 conventional dual-cure resin cements. The investigators concluded that although the bonding effectiveness of self-adhesive cements seems promising, their interaction with root dentin might be too weak to minimize microleakage at the post-cement-dentin interface.[142] In another study by Vrochari and coworkers, the degree of cure of 4 self-etching or self-adhesive resin cements in their self-curing mode was very low. The values obtained in the dual-curing mode were also low.[143]

Self-adhesive cements offer a new, simpler approach, but the efficacy of many recently marketed products is not known, and there are few data in the literature regarding their in vitro or clinical performance. At this point in their development, the literature generally shows them to be inferior to the total-etch method.

THE POST/RESIN INTERFACE

In addition to the interface between the resin cement and dentin, the post/resin interface is also important. Several surface treatments of the post have been recommended for improving the bonding of resin cements or core materials to fiber posts.

Silane Application

The literature is mixed on the value of application of silane to fiber posts. In one study, pretreatment of fiber posts with silane did not result in an enhanced bonding between post and 6 different resin cements[144] and the effect of silanization was reported to be clinically negligible.[145,146] Perdigão and colleagues[147] showed that the use of a silane coupling agent did not increase the push-out bond strengths of 3 different fiber posts. On the contrary, Goracci and colleagues[148] reported an improvement in bond strength between silanized fiber posts and flowable composite cores. Aksornmuang and colleagues[149] similarly confirmed the benefit of silane application in enhancing the microtensile bond strength of a dual-cure resin core material to translucent fiber posts.

Air Abrasion

It is well accepted that sandblasting with alumina particles results in an increased surface roughness and surface area, but it also provided mixed results when used with fiber posts. A study by Valandro and colleagues[150] showed that air abrasion with silica-coated aluminum oxide particles, followed by silanization, improved the bond strength between quartz fiber posts and resin cements. Sandblasting was also shown to improve the retention of fiber posts in 2 other studies.[151,152] The mechanical action of sandblasting probably removes of the superficial layer of resinous matrix, creating micro-retentive spaces on the post surface. On the other hand, Bitter and colleagues[144] reported little influence of sandblasting on the bond strength between fiber posts and resinous cements. Sahafi and colleagues[106] evaluated the efficacy of sand blasting the surface of zirconium and fiber posts with silica oxide. Despite the satisfactory bond strengths, the treatment was considered too aggressive for fiber posts, with the risk of significantly modifying their shape and fit within the root canals. Air abrasion should be used with caution, as it is difficult to standardize the procedure.

Alternative Etching Techniques

Hydrogen peroxide and sodium ethoxide are commonly employed for conditioning epoxy resin surfaces. The etching effect of these chemicals depends on partial resinous matrix dissolution, breaking epoxy resin bonds through substrate oxidation.[153] A similar approach has been proposed for pretreatment of fiber posts to increase their responsiveness to silanization, achieving satisfactory results for both chemicals.[154,155] The conditioning treatment consisted of fiber posts immersion in the solutions for 10 to 20 minutes. By removing a surface layer of epoxy resin, a larger surface area of exposed quartz fibers is available for silanization. The spaces between these fibers provide additional sites for micromechanical retention of the resin composites. Similar results were obtained by pretreating methacrylate-based posts with either hydrogen peroxide or hydrofluoric acid.[156]

Pretreatment with 24% H_2O_2 for 10 minutes, followed by silane application, seems to be a clinically feasible, inexpensive, and effective method for enhancing interfacial strengths between both methacrylate-based and epoxy resin-based fiber posts and resin composites.[155,156] Pretreatment with H_2O_2 can be performed well in advance of the clinical use.

CLINICAL PROCEDURES FOR FIBER POST CEMENTATION AND CORE BUILDUP

As discussed earlier, there are a lot of advantages to immediate post placement after finishing the endodontic treatment. The use of rubber dam, magnification, and good illumination are essential to carry out root canal treatment to a consistently high standard. Similar conditions are also required for all clinical procedures involving an adhesive bonding.

Gutta-percha can be removed with the aid of heat or chemicals, but most often the easiest and most efficient method is with rotary instruments. If the clinician who has performed the root canal treatment is going to place the post as well, obturation can be completed only in the apical portion of the canal.

There is a direct correlation between the diameter of the fiber post and fracture strength.[157] Büttel and colleagues[113] showed that post fit did not have a significant influence on fracture resistance, irrespective of the post length. Their results suggest that excessive post space preparation aimed at producing an optimal circumferential post fit is not required to improve fracture resistance of roots.

All remnants of gutta-percha, Resilon, sealer, and temporary filling materials should be removed using small micro-brushes with alcohol or a detergent. Acid-etching of the post space and an EDTA irrigation combined with ultrasonics are effective in obtaining a clean post space.[134,135] Air abrasion is an effective way the clean the pulp floor.

The use of a matrix helps confine the core material, enhances the adaptation of the composite to the remaining tooth structure and post, and prevents bonding core material to adjacent teeth. However, the use of a matrix is not essential.[158]

As discussed earlier, the use of a fourth-generation, 3-step etch-and-rinse adhesive with self-cure and dual-cure composites is recommended. If a self-etching adhesive is used, no rinsing takes place, which might result in dentin walls that are less clean. Moreover, when using a ZOE sealer, a self-etching adhesive incorporates Eugenol in the hybrid layer, which inhibits the polymerization of resins. After the etch-and-rinse step, paper points are recommended to dry the canal before the application of the primer and adhesive. The use of small micro-brushes has been shown to promote higher bond strength values than other brushes tested.[159] In the same study, the use of paper points to remove excess adhesive resulted in higher bond strengths.

A self-cure or dual-cure resin composite may be used rather than a separate luting cement for cementation of the post and the subsequent buildup. These composites may be bulk-filled because they do not require deep penetration with a curing light. Self-cure and dual-cure composites polymerize more slowly than light-cure materials, allowing the material to flow during polymerization contraction, and placing less stress on the adhesive bond.[24]

To minimize void formation, the composite is injected into the conditioned post channel using a syringe with a specially designed small tip, a so-called needle tube. The tip is inserted until it reaches the coronal part of the root canal filling, and is then applied from the base of the post channel coronally until the post space is filled to the brim. Then the pretreated post is immediately inserted into the composite filling the post space, without the need to further cover the post itself with composite. Finally, the composite core is added to the newly placed post, using the same self-cure or dual-cure composite applied into the post space. This procedure can be done immediately or after the composite in the post channel has completely set. A

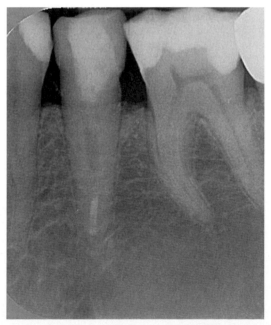

Fig. 7. Mandibular second premolar is treatment planned for an endodontic retreatment, post, core, and crown.

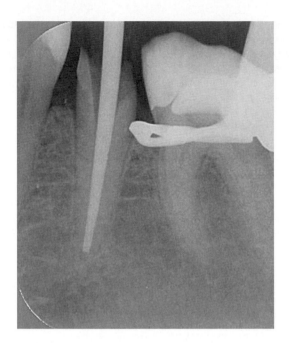

Fig. 8. Cone-fit.

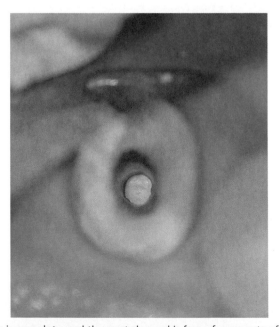

Fig. 9. Obturation is complete and the post channel is free of remnants of root canal filling. The obturating material is seen at the base of the post channel.

light-cured composite may also be used for the buildup. It is critical that the post is fully embedded in composite to avoid the uptake of moisture, which may compromise its mechanical properties.[160-162] Embedding can be obtained by cutting back the post a few millimeters below the cavo-surface margin before placement or after the composite of the core has completely set. If a matrix has been used, the core needs to be contoured and the occlusion needs to be adjusted. Another option is to complete the crown preparation at the same session.

CLINICAL SEQUENCE

1. Isolate the tooth with rubber dam and carry out root canal treatment (**Figs. 7** and **8**).
2. Remove all remnants of root filling and temporary filling materials using small micro-brushes with alcohol (**Fig. 9**).
3. Clean the floor with air abrasion.
4. Select a post that passively fits into the available canal space (**Fig. 10**).
5. Pre-fit the post and cut it back at the coronal or apical end to accommodate the existing post channel. In oval shaped canals, or premolars with 2 canals, consider placing 2 posts.
6. Confirm the fit of the post with a radiograph if necessary.
7. Air abrade the post surface with 50-μm alumina particles for 5 seconds, or use a pretreated post that has been immersed in 24% H_2O_2 for 10 minutes. Clean the post surface by acid-etching the surface with 37% phosphoric acid, rinse and air-dry.
8. Apply silane to the post surface according to the manufacturer's instructions.

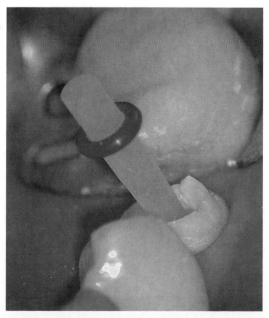

Fig. 10. The largest post that fits passively in the available post space is selected. After finishing the root canal treatment, no additional dentin is removed to accommodate the post.

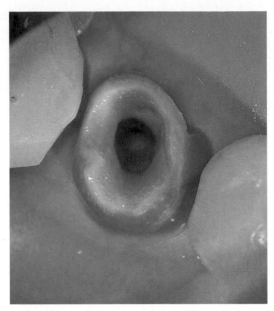

Fig. 11. Phosphoric acid 37% is applied to the dentin of the post channel and the remaining tooth structure.

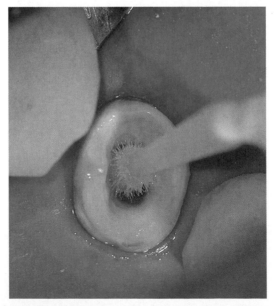

Fig. 12. The use of a small micro-brush greatly facilitates the application of dentin primer and adhesive into the post channel.

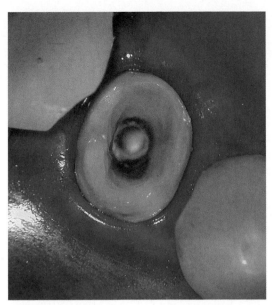

Fig. 13. A shiny surface confirms an even distribution of the dentin adhesive.

9. Acid-etch the enamel (if present) with 37% phosphoric acid for 30 seconds, and dentin for 15 seconds (**Fig. 11**).
10. Rinse and air-dry.
11. Use a small micro-brush to apply a primer that can be used with a self-cure or dual-cure core material to the dentin according to the manufacturer's instructions (**Fig. 12**). Gently air-dry.

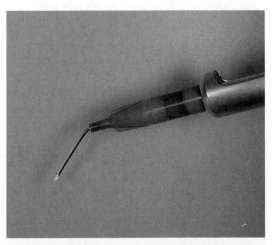

Fig. 14. The use of a needle tube for delivering composite into the post space minimizes void formation. The tip of the needle tube is inserted until it reaches the root canal filling. Then the composite is applied from the base of the post channel coronally, and the post space is filled to the brim. The post is immediately inserted into the composite.

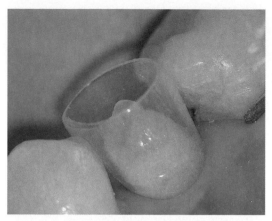

Fig. 15. A composite core is added to the newly placed post. To prevent bonding core material to adjacent teeth, as well as to enhance the adaptation of the composite to the remaining tooth structure, a core form is used as a matrix.

12. Apply a self-cure or dual-cure dental adhesive that can be used with a self-cure or dual-cure core material to the dentin according to the manufacturer's instructions (**Fig. 13**).
13. Inject a self-cure or dual-cure composite in the post space by using a needle tube (**Fig. 14**).
14. Insert the post into the post channel filled with composite.
15. Use a matrix to prevent bonding core material to adjacent teeth, as well as to enhance the adaptation of the composite to the remaining tooth structure (**Fig. 15**).

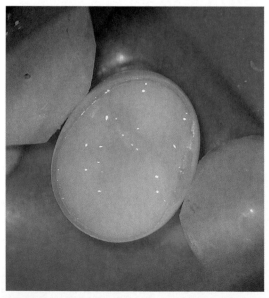

Fig. 16. The composite core is added to the newly placed post in a bulk fill, using the same self-curing composite placed in the post channel.

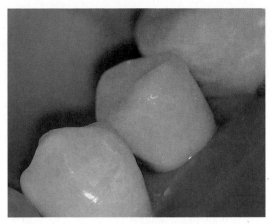

Fig. 17. The composite core is contoured and finished.

16. Add the remaining composite to the newly placed post or use a light-cure composite for that purpose in increments (**Fig. 16**).
17. Light-cure if necessary, or wait for at least 5 minutes until the self-cure composite has completely set.
18. Contour and adjust the occlusion (**Fig. 17**).
19. Finish and polish the restoration.
20. Take a final radiograph (**Fig. 18**).

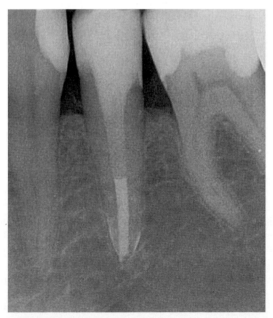

Fig. 18. The radiograph shows a well-adapted fiber post and composite buildup without voids, which is ready to be prepared for a crown.

SUMMARY AND RECOMMENDATIONS

- Evaluate restorability carefully before considering endodontic and restorative treatment.
- Preserve radicular and coronal dentin, especially in the cervical area, to maximize the long-term restorative result.
- Use adhesive procedures at both radicular and coronal levels to strengthen remaining tooth structure and optimize restoration stability and retention.
- Use post and core materials with physical properties similar to those of natural dentin.
- Use a rubber dam when performing clinical procedures involving adhesive bonding.
- Choose a post that fits passively into the canal preparation.
- Preserve an apical root canal filling of at least 4 to 5 mm.
- Use a post length that equals at least the crown height, and that extends apically beyond the crest of bone.
- Consider placing 2 posts in oval-shaped canals.
- Consider placing a fiber post through the existing crown in bridge abutments or small teeth. The post will increase crown retention and may improve resistance to fracture as long as no additional radicular dentin is removed in the process.
- With an adequate ferrule and canal thickness, use a fiber post to distribute forces more evenly in the root and reduce the chances of root fracture.
- If there is an inadequate ferrule, longevity may be compromised, no matter which post is used.
  - Metal posts are stronger and more resistant to flexure, but the stress distribution is unfavorable, with higher risk of root fracture.
  - The stress distribution in fiber posts is more favorable, but these posts are more susceptible to fracture and more likely to flex under load, which may result in micro-movements of the core, and subsequent leakage, caries, and retention loss.

REFERENCES

1. Kakehashi S, Stanley HR, Fitzgerald RJ. The effects of surgical exposures of dental pulps in germ-free and conventional laboratory rats. Oral Surg Oral Med Oral Pathol 1965;20:340–9.
2. Siqueira JF Jr. Aetiology of root canal treatment failure and why well-treated teeth can fail. Int Endod J 2001;34:1–10.
3. Saunders WP, Saunders EM. Coronal leakage as a cause of failure in root canal therapy: a review. Endod Dent Traumatol 1994;10:105–8.
4. Alves J, Walton R, Drake D. Coronal leakage: endotoxin penetration from mixed bacterial communities through obturated, post-prepared root canals. J Endod 1998;24:587–91.
5. Ray HA, Trope M. Periapical status of endodontically treated teeth in relation to the technical quality of the root filling and the coronal restoration. Int Endod J 1995;28:12–8.
6. Iqbal MK, Johansson AA, Akeel RF, et al. A retrospective analysis of factors associated with the periapical status of restored, endodontically treated teeth. Int J Prosthodont 2003;16(1):31–8.

7. Willershausen B, Tekyatan H, Krummenauer F, et al. Survival rate of endodontically treated teeth in relation to conservative vs post insertion techniques— a retrospective study. Eur J Med Res 2005;10(5):204–8.
8. Ferrari M, Cagidiaco MC, Goracci C, et al. Long-term retrospective study of the clinical performance of fiber posts. Am J Dent 2007;20(5):287–91.
9. Creugers NH, Mentink AG, Fokkinga WA, et al. 5-year follow-up of a prospective clinical study on various types of core restorations. Int J Prosthodont 2005;18(1): 34–9.
10. Fokkinga WA, Le Bell AM, Kreulen CM, et al. Ex vivo fracture resistance of direct resin composite complete crowns with and without posts on maxillary premolars. Int Endod J 2005;38(4):230–7.
11. Buonocore MG. A simple method of increasing the adhesion of acrylic filling materials to enamel surfaces. J Dent Res 1955;34(6):849–53.
12. Van Meerbeek B, De Munck J, Yoshida Y, et al. Buonocore memorial lecture. Adhesion to enamel and dentin: current status and future challenges. Oper Dent 2003;28(3):215–35.
13. Tagami J, Hosoda H, Fusayama T. Optimal technique of etching enamel. Oper Dent 1988;13(4):181–4.
14. Fabianelli A, Kugel G, Ferrari M. Efficacy of self-etching primer on sealing margins of Class II restorations. Am J Dent 2003;16(1):37–41.
15. De Munck J, Van Meerbeek B, Yoshida Y, et al. Four-year water degradation of total-etch adhesives bonded to dentin. J Dent Res 2003;82(2):136–40.
16. Knight JS, Holmes JR, Bradford H, et al. Shear bond strengths of composite bonded to porcelain using porcelain repair systems. Am J Dent 2003;16(4): 252–4.
17. Kato H, Matsumura H, Tanaka T, et al. Bond strength and durability of porcelain bonding systems. J Prosthet Dent 1996;75(2):163–8.
18. Pashley DH. Smear layer: overview of structure and function. Proc Finn Dent Soc 1992;88(Suppl 1):215–24.
19. Pashley DH, Tao L, Boyd L, et al. Scanning electron microscopy of the substructure of smear layers in human dentine. Arch Oral Biol 1988;33:265–70.
20. Mjor IA, Sveen OB, Heyeraas KJ. Pulp-dentin biology in restorative dentistry. Part 1: normal structure and physiology. Quintessence Int 2001;32:427–46.
21. Nakabayashi N, Kojima K, Masuhara E. The promotion of adhesion by the infiltration of monomers into tooth substrates. J Biomed Mater Res 1982;16:265–73.
22. Okuda M, Pereira PN, Nakajima M, et al. Long-term durability of resin dentin interface: nanoleakage vs. microtensile bond strength. Oper Dent 2002;27(3): 289–96.
23. Carvalho RM, Pereira JC, Yoshiyama M, et al. A review of polymerization contraction: the influence of stress development versus stress relief. Oper Dent 1996;21(1):17–24.
24. Braga RR, Ferracane JL. Alternatives in polymerization contraction stress management. Crit Rev Oral Biol Med 2004;15:176–84.
25. Braga RR, Ballester RY, Ferracane JL. Factors involved in the development of polymerization shrinkage stress in resin-composites: a systematic review. Dent Mater 2005;21:962–70.
26. Braga RR, Ferracane JL, Condon JR. Polymerization contraction stress in dual-cure cements and its effect on interfacial integrity of bonded inlays. J Dent 2002; 30(7–8):333–40.
27. Feilzer AJ, de Gee AJ, Davidson CL. Increased wall-to-wall curing contraction in thin bonded resin layers. J Dent Res 1989;68:48–50.

28. Alster D, Feilzer AJ, de Gee AJ, et al. Polymerization contraction stress in thin resin composite layers as a function of layer thickness. Dent Mater 1997; 13(3):146–50.
29. Shirai K, De Munck J, Yoshida Y, et al. Effect of cavity configuration and aging on the bonding effectiveness of six adhesives to dentin. Dent Mater 2005;21(2): 110–24.
30. De Munck J, Van Landuyt K, Peumans M, et al. A critical review of the durability of adhesion to tooth tissue: methods and results. J Dent Res 2005;84(2):118–32.
31. de Oliveira Carrilho MR, Tay FR, Pashley DH, et al. Mechanical stability of resin-dentin bond components. Dent Mater 2005;21(3):232–41.
32. Hashimoto M, Ohno H, Kaga M, et al. In vivo degradation of resin-dentin bonds in humans over 1 to 3 years. J Dent Res 2000;79(6):1385–91.
33. Hashimoto M, Ohno H, Kaga M, et al. Resin-tooth adhesive interfaces after long-term function. Am J Dent 2001;14(4):211–5.
34. Okuda M, Pereira PN, Nakajima M, et al. Relationship between nanoleakage and long-term durability of dentin bonds. Oper Dent 2001;26(5):482–90.
35. Frankenberger R, Pashley DH, Reich SM, et al. Characterisation of resin-dentine interfaces by compressive cyclic loading. Biomaterials 2005;26(14):2043–52.
36. Tay FR, Loushine RJ, Lambrechts P, et al. Geometric factors affecting dentin bonding in root canals: a theoretical modeling approach. J Endod 2005;31(8):584–9.
37. Davidson CL, de Gee AJ. Relaxation of polymerization contraction stress by flow in dental composites. J Dent Res 1984;63:146–8.
38. Yoshikawa T, Sano H, Burrow MF, et al. Effects of dentin depth and cavity configuration on bond strength. J Dent Res 1999;78(4):898–905.
39. Hannig M, Friedrichs C. Comparative in vivo and in vitro investigation of interfacial bond variability. Oper Dent 2001;26(1):3–11.
40. Tay FR, Loushine RJ, Weller RN, et al. Ultrastructural evaluation of the apical seal in roots filled with a polycaprolactone-based root canal filling material. J Endod 2005;31(7):514–9.
41. Goracci C, Fabianelli A, Sadek FT, et al. The contribution of friction to the dislocation resistance of bonded fiber posts. J Endod 2005;31(8):608–12.
42. Pirani C, Chersoni S, Foschi F, et al. Does hybridization of intraradicular dentin really improve fiber post retention in endodontically treated teeth? J Endod 2005;31(12):891–4.
43. Roulet JF. Marginal integrity: clinical significance. J Dent 1994;22(Suppl 1): S9–12.
44. Tay FR, Pashley DH, Yoshiyama M. Two modes of nanoleakage expression in single-step adhesives. J Dent Res 2002;81(7):472–6.
45. Bouillaguet S, Troesch S, Wataha JC, et al. Microtensile bond strength between adhesive cements and root canal dentin. Dent Mater 2003;19(3):199–205.
46. Tay FR, Pashley DH, Yiu CK, et al. Factors contributing to the incompatibility between simplified-step adhesives and chemically-cured or dual-cured composites. Part I. Single-step self-etching adhesive. J Adhes Dent 2003; 5(1):27–40.
47. Tay FR, Suh BI, Pashley DH, et al. Factors contributing to the incompatibility between simplified-step adhesives and self-cured or dual-cured composites. Part II. Single-bottle, total-etch adhesive. J Adhes Dent 2003;5(2):91–105.
48. Lai SC, Mak YF, Cheung GS, et al. Reversal of compromised bonding to oxidized etched dentin. J Dent Res 2001;80(10):1919–24.
49. Ari H, Yasar E, Belli S. Effects of NaOCl on bond strengths of resin cements to root canal dentin. J Endod 2003;29(4):248–51.

50. Erdemir A, Ari H, Gungunes H, et al. Effect of medications for root canal treatment on bonding to root canal dentin. J Endod 2004;30(2):113–6.
51. Yiu CK, Garcia-Godoy F, Tay FR, et al. A nanoleakage perspective on bonding to oxidized dentin. J Dent Res 2002;81(9):628–32.
52. Doyle MD, Loushine RJ, Agee KA, et al. Improving the performance of EndoRez root canal sealer with a dual-cured two-step self-etch adhesive. I. Adhesive strength to dentin. J Endod 2006;32(8):766–70.
53. Sorensen JA, Martinoff JT. Intracoronal reinforcement and coronal coverage: a study of endodontically treated teeth. J Prosthet Dent 1984;51(6):780–4.
54. Cheung GS, Chan TK. Long-term survival of primary root canal treatment carried out in a dental teaching hospital. Int Endod J 2003;36:117–28.
55. Salehrabi R, Rotstein I. Endodontic treatment outcomes in a large patient population in the USA: an epidemiological study. J Endod 2004;30(12):846–50.
56. Aquilino SA, Caplan DJ. Relationship between crown placement and the survival of endodontically treated teeth. J Prosthet Dent 2002;87(3):256–63.
57. Nagasiri R, Chitmongkolsuk S. Long-term survival of endodontically treated molars without crown coverage: a retrospective cohort study. J Prosthet Dent 2005;93(2):164–70.
58. Fokkinga WA, Kreulen CM, Bronkhorst EM, et al. Up to 17-year controlled clinical study on post-and-cores and covering crowns. J Dent 2007;35(10):778–86.
59. Sorensen JA, Engelman MJ. Ferrule design and fracture resistance of endodontically treated teeth. J Prosthet Dent 1990;63(5):529–36.
60. Isidor F, Brøndum K, Ravnholt G. The influence of post length and crown ferrule length on the resistance to cyclic loading of bovine teeth with prefabricated titanium posts. Int J Prosthodont 1999;12:78–82.
61. Stankiewicz N, Wilson P. The ferrule effect. Dent Update 2008;35(4):222–4, 227–8.
62. Zhi-Yue L, Yu-Xing Z. Effects of post-core design and ferrule on fracture resistance of endodontically treated maxillary central incisors. J Prosthet Dent 2003;89:368–73.
63. Ng CC, Dumbrigue HB, Al-Bayat MI, et al. Influence of remaining coronal tooth structure location on the fracture resistance of restored endodontically treated anterior teeth. J Prosthet Dent 2006;95(4):290–6.
64. Goodacre CJ, Spolnik KJ. The prosthodontic management of endodontically treated teeth: a literature review. Part I. Success and failure data, treatment concepts. J Prosthodont 1994;3(4):243–50.
65. Balto H, Al-Nazhan S, Al-Mansour K, et al. Microbial leakage of Cavit, IRM, and Temp Bond in post-prepared root canals using two methods of gutta-percha removal: an in vitro study. J Contemp Dent Pract 2005;6(3):53–61.
66. Ricketts DN, Tait CM, Higgins AJ. Tooth preparation for post-retained restorations. Br Dent J 2005;198(8):463–71.
67. Hunter AJ, Feiglin B, Williams JF. Effects of post placement on endodontically treated teeth. J Prosthet Dent 1989;62(2):166–72.
68. Heydecke G, Butz F, Strub JR. Fracture strength and survival rate of endodontically treated maxillary incisors with approximal cavities after restoration with different post and core systems: an in vitro study. J Dent 2001;29:427–33.
69. Kuttler S, McLean A, Dorn S, et al. The impact of post space preparation with Gates-Glidden drills on residual dentin thickness in distal roots of mandibular molars. J Am Dent Assoc 2004;135(7):903–9.
70. Fennis WM, Kuijs RH, Kreulen CM, et al. A survey of cusp fractures in a population of general dental practices. Int J Prosthodont 2002;15(6):559–63.

71. De Backer H, Van Maele G, Decock V, et al. Long-term survival of complete crowns, fixed dental prostheses, and cantilever fixed dental prostheses with posts and cores on root canal-treated teeth. Int J Prosthodont 2007;20(3):229–34.

72. Guzy GE, Nichols JI. In vitro comparison of intact endodontically treated teeth with and without endo-post reinforcement. J Prosthet Dent 1979;42:39–44.

73. Trope M, Maltz DO, Tronstad L. Resistance to fracture of restored endodontically treated teeth. Endod Dent Traumatol 1985;1:108–11.

74. Schmitter M, Huy C, Ohlmann B, et al. Fracture resistance of upper and lower incisors restored with glass fiber reinforced posts. J Endod 2006;32(4):328–30.

75. Rosentritt M, Sikora M, Behr M, et al. In vitro fracture resistance and marginal adaptation of metallic and tooth-coloured post systems. J Oral Rehabil 2004; 31(7):675–81.

76. Salameh Z, Sorrentino R, Ounsi HF, et al. Effect of different all-ceramic crown system on fracture resistance and failure pattern of endodontically treated maxillary premolars restored with and without glass fiber posts. J Endod 2007;33(7):848–51.

77. Carvalho CA, Valera MC, Oliveira LD, et al. Structural resistance in immature teeth using root reinforcements in vitro. Dent Traumatol 2005;21(3):155–9.

78. Goncalves LA, Vansan LP, Paulino SM, et al. Fracture resistance of weakened roots restored with a transilluminating post and adhesive restorative materials. J Prosthet Dent 2006;96(5):339–44.

79. Hayashi M, Takahashi Y, Imazato S, et al. Fracture resistance of pulpless teeth restored with post-cores and crowns. Dent Mater 2006;22(5):477–85.

80. D'Arcangelo C, De Angelis F, Vadini M, et al. In vitro fracture resistance and deflection of pulpless teeth restored with fiber posts and prepared for veneers. J Endod 2008;34(7):838–41.

81. Salameh Z, Sorrentino R, Ounsi HF, et al. The effect of different full-coverage crown systems on fracture resistance and failure pattern of endodontically treated maxillary incisors restored with and without glass fiber posts. J Endod 2008;34(7):842–6.

82. Naumann M, Preuss A, Frankenberger R. Reinforcement effect of adhesively luted fiber reinforced composite versus titanium posts. Dent Mater 2007;23(2):138–44.

83. Abdul Salam SN, Banerjee A, Mannocci F, et al. Cyclic loading of endodontically treated teeth restored with glass fibre and titanium alloy posts: fracture resistance and failure modes. Eur J Prosthodont Restor Dent 2006;14(3): 98–104.

84. Krejci I, Duc O, Dietschi D, et al. Marginal adaptation, retention and fracture resistance of adhesive composite restorations on devitalized teeth with and without posts. Oper Dent 2003;28:127–35.

85. Duret B, Reynaud M, Duret F. New concept of coronoradicular reconstruction: the Composipost (1). Chir Dent Fr 1990;60(540):131–41.

86. Standlee JP, Caputo AA, Hanson EC. Retention of endodontic dowels: effects of cement, dowel length, diameter, and design. J Prosthet Dent 1978;39:401–5.

87. Martinez-Insua A, da Silva L, Rilo B, et al. Comparison of the fracture resistances of pulpless teeth restored with a cast post and core or carbon-fiber post with a composite core. J Prosthet Dent 1998;80:527–32.

88. Standlee JP, Caputo AA. The retentive and stress distributing properties of split threaded endodontic dowels. J Prosthet Dent 1992;68:436–42.

89. Mannocci F, Ferrari M, Watson TF. Intermittent loading of teeth restoredusing quartz fiber, carbon-quartz fiber, and zirconium dioxide ceramic root canal posts. J Adhes Dent 1999;1:153–8.

90. Akkayan B, Gülmez T. Resistance to fracture of endodontically treated teeth restored with different post systems. J Prosthet Dent 2002;87(4):431–7.
91. Fokkinga WA, Kreulen CM, Vallittu PK, et al. A structured analysis of in vitro failure loads and failure modes of fiber, metal, and ceramic post-and-core systems. Int J Prosthodont 2004;17(4):476–82.
92. Butz F, Lennon AM, Heydecke G, et al. Survival rate and fracture strength of endodontically treated maxillary incisors with moderate defects restored with different post-and-core systems: an in vitro study. Int J Prosthodont 2001;14: 58–64.
93. Ottl P, Hahn L, Lauer HC, et al. Fracture characteristics of carbon fibre, ceramic and non-palladium endodontic post systems at monotonously increasing loads. J Oral Rehabil 2002;29:175–83.
94. Kivanç BH, Görgül G. Fracture resistance of teeth restored with different post systems using new-generation adhesives. J Contemp Dent Pract 2008;9(7): 33–40.
95. Dietschi D, Duc O, Krejci I, et al. Biomechanical considerations for the restoration of endodontically treated teeth: a systematic review of the literature, Part 1. Composition and micro- and macrostructure alterations. Quintessence Int 2007; 38(9):733–43.
96. Maccari PC, Conceicao EN, Nunes MF. Fracture resistance of endodontically treated teeth restored with three different prefabricated esthetic posts. J Esthet Restor Dent 2003;15(1):25–30.
97. Newman MP, Yaman P, Dennison J, et al. Fracture resistance of endodontically treated teeth restored with composite posts. J Prosthet Dent 2003;89:360–7.
98. Cagidiaco MC, Goracci C, Garcia-Godoy F, et al. Clinical studies of fiber posts: a literature review. Int J Prosthodont 2008;21(4):328–36.
99. Signore A, Benedicenti S, Kaitsas V, et al. Long-term survival of endodontically treated, maxillary anterior teeth restored with either tapered or parallel-sided glass-fiber posts and full-ceramic crown coverage. J Dent 2009;37(2):115–21.
100. Ferrari M, Vichi A, Garcia-Godoy F. Clinical evaluation of fiber-reinforced epoxy-resin posts and cast posts and cores. Am J Dent 2000;13:15B–8B.
101. Dietschi D, Duc O, Krejci I, et al. Biomechanical considerations for the restoration of endodontically treated teeth: a systematic review of the literature, Part II (Evaluation of fatigue behavior, interfaces, and in vivo studies). Quintessence Int 2008;39(2):117–29.
102. Sundh B, Odman P. A study of fixed prosthodontics performed at a university clinic 18 years after insertion. Int J Prosthodont 1997;10(6):513–9.
103. Morgano SM, Brackett SE. Foundation restorations in fixed prosthodontics: current knowledge and future needs. J Prosthet Dent 1999;82(6):643–57.
104. Drummond JL. In vitro evaluation of endodontic posts. Am J Dent 2000;13(Spec No):5B–8B.
105. Drummond JL, Bapna MS. Static and cyclic loading of fiber-reinforced dental resin. Dent Mater 2003;19:226–31.
106. Lassila LV, Tanner J, Le Bell AM, et al. Flexural properties of fiber reinforced root canal posts. Dent Mater 2004;20(1):29–36.
107. Sahafi A, Peutzfeldt A, Asmussen E, et al. Retention and failure morphology of prefabricated posts. Int J Prosthodont 2004;17(3):307–12.
108. Teixeira EC, Teixeira FB, Piasick JR, et al. An in vitro assessment of prefabricated fiber post systems. J Am Dent Assoc 2006;137(7):1006–12.
109. Perdigao J, Geraldeli S, Lee IK. Push-out bond strengths of tooth-colored posts bonded with different adhesive systems. Am J Dent 2004;17(6):422–6.

110. Sadek FT, Boracci C, Monticelli F, et al. Immediate and 24-hour evaluation of the interfacial strengths of fiber posts. J Endod 2006;32(12):1174–7.
111. Goracci C, Tavares AU, Fabianelli A, et al. The adhesion between fiber posts and root canal walls: comparison between microtensile and push-out bond strength measurements. Eur J Oral Sci 2004;112(4):353–61.
112. Braga NM, Paulino SM, Alfredo E, et al. Removal resistance of glass-fiber and metallic cast posts with different lengths. J Oral Sci 2006;48(1):15–20.
113. Büttel L, Krastl G, Lorch H, et al. Influence of post fit and post length on fracture resistance. Int Endod J 2009;42(1):47–53.
114. Innella R, Autieri G, Ceruti P, et al. Relation between length of fiber post and its mechanical retention. Minerva Stomatol 2005;54(9):481–8.
115. Adanir N, Belli S. Evaluation of different post lengths' effect on fracture resistance of a glass fiber post system. Eur J Dent 2008;2(1):23–8.
116. Kvist T, Rydin E, Reit C. The relative frequency of periapical lesions in teeth with root canal-retained posts. J Endod 1989;15(12):578–80.
117. Wu MK, Pehlivan Y, Kontakiotis EG, et al. Microleakage along apical root fillings and cemented posts. J Prosthet Dent 1998;79(3):264–9.
118. Abramovitz I, Tagger M, Tamse A, et al. The effect of immediate vs. delayed post space preparation on the apical seal of a root canal filling: a study in an increased-sensitivity pressure-driven system. J Endod 2000;26(8):435–9.
119. Lui JL. Depth of composite polymerization within simulated root canals using light-transmitting posts. Oper Dent 1994;19(5):165–8.
120. Roberts HW, Leonard DL, Vandewalle KS, et al. The effect of a translucent post on resin composite depth of cure. Dent Mater 2004;20:617–22.
121. Yoldas O, Alaçam T. Microhardness of composites in simulated root canals cured with light transmitting posts and glass-fiber reinforced composite posts. J Endod 2005;31:104–6.
122. Faria e Silva AL, Arias VG, Soares LE, et al. Influence of fiber-post translucency on the degree of conversion of a dual-cured resin cement. J Endod 2007;33(3):303–5.
123. Goracci C, Corciolani G, Vichi A, et al. Light-transmitting ability of marketed fiber posts. J Dent Res 2008;87(12):1122–6.
124. dos Santos Alves Morgan LF, Peixoto RT, de Castro Albuquerque R, et al. Light transmission through a translucent fiber post. J Endod 2008;34(3): 299–302.
125. Mulvay PG, Abbott PV. The effect of endodontic access cavity preparation and subsequent restorative procedures on molar crown retention. Aust Dent J 1996; 41(2):134–9.
126. Hachmeister KA, Dunn WJ, Murchison DF, et al. Fracture strength of amalgam crowns with repaired endodontic access. Oper Dent 2002;27(3):254–8.
127. Fan B, Wu MK, Wesselink PR. Coronal leakage along apical root fillings after immediate and delayed post spaces preparation. Endod Dent Traumatol 1999;15:124–7.
128. Solano F, Hartwell G, Appelstein C. Comparison of apical leakage between immediate versus delayed post space preparation using AH Plus sealer. J Endod 2005;31(10):752–4.
129. Dalat DM, Spångberg LS. Effect of post preparation on the apical seal of teeth obturated with plastic thermafil obturators. Oral Surg Oral Med Oral Pathol 1993; 76(6):760–5.
130. Vano M, Cury AH, Goracci C, et al. The effect of immediate versus delayed cementation on the retention of different types of fiber post in canals obturated using a eugenol sealer. J Endod 2006;32(9):882–5.

131. Vano M, Cury AH, Goracci C, et al. Retention of fiber posts cemented at different time intervals in canals obturated using an epoxy resin sealer. J Dent 2008; 36(10):801–7.
132. Hagge MS, Wong RD, Lindemuth JS. Retention strengths of five luting cements on prefabricated dowels after root canal obturation with a zinc oxide/eugenol sealer: 1. Dowel space preparation/cementation at one week after obturation. J Prosthodont 2002;11(3):168–75.
133. Serafino C, Gallina G, Cumbo E, et al. Surface debris of canal walls after post space preparation in endodontically treated teeth: a scanning electron microscopic study. Oral Surg Oral Med Oral Pathol Oral Radiol Endod 2004;97(3):381–7.
134. Coniglio I, Magni E, Goracci C, et al. Post space cleaning using a new nickel titanium endodontic drill combined with different cleaning regimens. J Endod 2008;34(1):83–6.
135. Zhang L, Huang L, Xiong Y, et al. Effect of post-space treatment on retention of fiber posts in different root regions using two self-etching systems. Eur J Oral Sci 2008;116(3):280–6.
136. Fox K, Gutteridge DL. An in vitro study of coronal microleakage in root canal treated teeth restored by the post and core technique. Int Endod J 1997;30: 361–8.
137. Demarchi MGA, Sato EFL. Leakage of interim post and cores used during laboratory fabrication of custom posts. J Endod 2002;28:328–9.
138. Goracci C, Sadek FT, Fabianelli A, et al. Evaluation of the adhesion of fiber posts to intraradicular dentin. Oper Dent 2005;30(5):627–35.
139. Valandro LF, Filho OD, Valcra MC, et al. The effect of adhesive systems on the pullout strength of a fiberglass-reinforced composite post system in bovine teeth. J Adhes Dent 2005;7(4):331–6.
140. Radovic I, Mazzitelli C, Chieffi N, et al. Evaluation of the adhesion of fiber posts cemented using different adhesive approaches. Eur J Oral Sci 2008;116(6): 557–63.
141. Lührs AK, Guhr S, Günay H, et al. Shear bond strength of self-adhesive resins compared to resin cements with etch and rinse adhesives to enamel and dentin in vitro. Clin Oral Investig 2009 May 9. [Epub ahead of print].
142. Zicari F, Couthino E, De Munck J, et al. Bonding effectiveness and sealing ability of fiber-post bonding. Dent Mater 2008;24(7):967–77.
143. Vrochari AD, Eliades G, Hellwig E, et al. Curing efficiency of four self-etching, self-adhesive resin cements. Dent Mater 2009;25(9):1104–8.
144. Bitter K, Meyer-Lückel H, Priehn K, et al. Bond strengths of resin cements to fiber-reinforced composite posts. Am J Dent 2006;19(3):138–42.
145. Bitter K, Noetzel J, Neumann K, et al. Effect of silanization on bond strengths of fiber posts to various resin cements. Quintessence Int 2007;38(2):121–8.
146. Wrbas KT, Altenburger MJ, Schirrmeister JF, et al. Effect of adhesive resin cements and post surface silanization on the bond strengths of adhesively inserted fiber posts. J Endod 2007;33(7):840–3.
147. Perdigão J, Gomes G, Lee IK. The effect of silane on the bond strengths of fiber posts. Dent Mater 2006;22(8):752–8.
148. Goracci C, Raffaelli O, Monticelli F, et al. The adhesion between prefabricated FRC posts and composite resincores: microtensile bond strength with and without post-silanization. Dent Mater 2005;21(5):437–44.
149. Aksornmuang J, Nakajima M, Foxton RM, et al. Regional bond strengths of a dual-cure resin core material to translucent quartz fiber post. Am J Dent 2006;19(1):51–5.

150. Valandro LF, Yoshiga S, De Melo RM, et al. Microtensile bond strength between a quartz fiberpost and a resin cement: effect of post surface conditioning. J Adhes Dent 2006;8(2):105–11.
151. Balbosh A, Kern M. Effect of surface treatment on retention of glassfiber endodontic posts. J Prosthet Dent 2006;95(3):218–23.
152. Radovic I, Monticelli F, Goracci C, et al. The effect of sandblasting on adhesion of a dual-cured resin composite to methacrylic fiber posts: microtensile bond strength and SEM evaluation. J Dent 2007;35(6):496–502.
153. Monticelli F, Osorio R, Sadek FT, et al. Surface treatments for improving bond strength to prefabricated fiber posts: a literature review. Oper Dent 2008; 33(3):346–55.
154. Monticelli F, Osorio R, Toledano M, et al. Improving the quality of the quartz fiber postcore bond using sodiumethoxide etching and combined silane/adhesive coupling. J Endod 2006;32(5):447–51.
155. Monticelli F, Toledano M, Tay FR, et al. A simple etching technique for improving the retention of fiber posts to resin composites. J Endod 2006;32(1):44–7.
156. Vano M, Goracci C, Monticelli F, et al. The adhesion between fibre posts and composite resin cores: the evaluation of microtensile bond strength following various surface chemical treatments to posts. Int Endod J 2006;39(1):31–9.
157. Amaral M, Favarin Santini M, Wandscher V, et al. Effect of coronal macroretentions and diameter of a glass-FRC on fracture resistance of bovine teeth restored with fiber posts. Minerva Stomatol 2009;58(3):99–106.
158. Monticelli F, Goracci C, Ferrari M. Micromorphology of the fiber post-resin core unit: a scanning electron microscopy evaluation. Dent Mater 2004;20(2):176–83.
159. Souza RO, Lombardo GH, Michida SM, et al. Influence of brush type as carrier of adhesive solutions and paper points as adhesive-excess remover on the resin bond to root canal dentin. J Adhes Dent 2007;9:521–6.
160. Mannoci F, Cavalli G, Gagliani M. Adhesive restoration of endodontically treated teeth. Endodontics 4. Quintessentials of Dental Practice, vol. 40. London: Quintessence Publishing Co Ltd; 2008.
161. Torbjorner A, Karlsson S, Syverud M, et al. Carbon fiber reinforced root canal posts. Mechanical and cytotoxic properties. Eur J Oral Sci 1996;104(5–6): 605–11.
162. Mannocci F, Sherriff M, Watson TF. Three-point bending test of fiber posts. J Esthet Restor Dent 2003;15(5):313–8.

Essentials of Endodontic Microsurgery

Stephen P. Niemczyk, DMD[a,b,c,d,e,*]

KEYWORDS

- Endodontic microsurgery • Ergonomics • Root end resection
- Root end preparation • Root end filling

In his book *Working in a Small Place* Mark Shelton chronicles the efforts of a young neurosurgeon, Dr Peter Jannetta, to introduce a radically new microsurgical technique for cranial nerve decompression. Pivotal to the technique was the use of the surgical operating microscope (SOM) for precise visualization and manipulation of the delicate structures. What Dr Jannetta discovered was that not only was the use of the SOM in neurosurgery a rare event but also this particular piece of armamentarium was regarded with disdain by the "Grand Old Men" of the profession. Programs were hesitant to implement this technology, and their residents were discouraged in its use because the senior staff members either felt estranged by the unfamiliarity with the SOM, or threatened by its presence. What Dr Jannetta realized was that, rather than trying to convince the grand old men of the merits of the SOM, he would work from within the system, slowly teaching his residents and wait for a new generation, his generation, to assume the role of senior staff members. He is quoted in the book as saying "It takes twenty years for anything new to really catch on, not because it takes that long to convince the establishment, but because it takes that long for there to be a changeover to people who have grown up with the new idea as being accepted."[1] Today, all residency programs in neurosurgery require proficiency with the SOM and microsurgery.

An interesting parallel is drawn when one examines the progression of the dental operating microscope (DOM) use in dentistry and, specifically, endodontics. Although

Movies can be viewed within this article at http://www.dental.theclinics.com, April 2010 issue.
a Post Graduate Endodontic Program, Harvard School of Dental Medicine, Boston, MA, USA
b Post Graduate Endodontic Program, Dental Division, Albert Einstein Medical Center, Philadelphia, PA, USA
c Graduate Endodontic Program, National Naval Medical Center, Bethesda, MD, USA
d United States Army Endodontic Program, Fort Gordon, GA, USA
e 5100 Township Line Road, Drexel Hill, PA 19026, USA
* 5100 Township Line Road, Drexel Hill, PA 19026.
E-mail address: spndo@comcast.net

Dent Clin N Am 54 (2010) 375–399
doi:10.1016/j.cden.2009.12.002
0011-8532/10/$ – see front matter © 2010 Elsevier Inc. All rights reserved.

presented as early as 1986 by Selden,[2] it was not until the early 1990s that the DOM was introduced to the profession and graduate-level endodontic programs.[3-6] The usefulness of the DOM in endodontics was viewed with similar skepticism by the senior attendings of most programs for all the same reasons of their counterparts in neurosurgery. However, a concerted effort was made by a few enlightened individuals with foresight enough to recognize the advantages that microscopy could afford, and they lobbied their cause until the late 1990s, when it was mandated that all graduate programs and students demonstrate a proficiency in the use of the DOM. Before 1999, only 52% of the endodontists surveyed reported using the DOM.[7] Compare that to a more recent survey,[8] in which the age of the operator was compared with their usage of the DOM and it was found that the younger respondents (35 years old or younger) used the DOM 97% of the time for surgical and nonsurgical treatment. It is clear that the recent graduates are not only more comfortable with its use, but are also more accustomed to rendering treatment with the DOM. What is an interesting coincidence is that endodontics is approaching the 20-year mark of the inception of the DOM into practice; it would seem that Dr Jannetta's prophecies extend to the dental profession as well!

Although the basic principles of endodontic surgery have not been dramatically changed, advances in armamentarium and microtechniques have attempted to keep pace with the demands of today's endodontic microsurgical environment: greater ergonomic flexibility, more efficient preparation and placement of the root end filling (REF), and more biocompatibility of the materials used.

ANESTHESIA AND HEMOSTASIS

These 2 facets are inexorably linked because the effectiveness of the surgeon's administration preoperatively not only influences the comfort of the patient during the procedure but also the control of hemorrhage at the surgical site. Standard protocol is divided into regional and local injections and are as follows:

1. The administration of a long-acting anesthetic agent such as bupivicaine (Marcaine) as a block technique to obtain a sustained level of anesthesia beyond the duration of the surgery. For posterior surgeries this entails, for maxillary sites, a posterior superior and middle superior alveolar block; for posterior mandibular sites, an inferior alveolar nerve block supplemented with a mental nerve trunk block. Maxillary anterior teeth are blocked using bilateral anterior superior alveolar or infraorbital injections, while mandibular anterior teeth receive bilateral mental nerve blocks. All of these can be supplemented, as need be, with corresponding palatal or lingual infiltrations of the same anesthetic.

In studies examining the effectiveness of lidocaine versus bupivicaine, it was shown that lidocaine was faster in onset of lip numbness while bupivicaine resulted in longer duration.[9] However, Gordon and colleagues[10] have shown that administration of bupivicaine following surgical extractions resulted in decreased pain for longer periods of time. By minimizing the peripheral barrage of peripheral nociceptive neurons, it reduced the development of central sensitization, thought to mediate partially the central component of allodynia and hyperalgesia. This postoperative effect can be further enhanced by the preoperative administration of a nonsteroidal anti-inflammatory drug, resulting in statistically less postoperative discomfort and delay of onset of pain.[11,12] This peripheral block should be allowed to take effect (8–10 minutes) and signs of adequate anesthesia noted before the next phase.

2. Once regional anesthesia has been achieved, then a local infiltration of lidocaine 1:50,000 epinephrine is injected over the intended flap extent, concentrating the bulk of the infiltration over the surgical site. The injection speed is slow and steady (1–2 min/mL), allowing time for diffusion of the fluid and avoiding the formation of a bolus accumulating in the submucosa.[13] Done correctly, blanching will be evident in the surrounding tissues, spreading throughout the flap and its perimeter. Care should be taken to avoid injecting into skeletal muscle. Doing so will activate the β-adrenergic receptors, triggering vasodilation instead of constriction, causing undue hemorrhage on flap reflection and subsequent limited visibility of the surgical site.[13,14]

The outlined protocol is, of course, predicated on the systemic health of the patient and their ability to tolerate not only the surgical stress but also the cardiovascular impact of the epinephrine in the selected anesthetic. Even in healthy patients a transient tachycardia of short duration is not uncommon, but is usually well tolerated if the patient has been forewarned. However, in cases where underlying cardiovascular diseases such as uncontrolled hypertension or history of recent cardiac surgery place these patients at a higher risk, the surgeon would be prudent to consult with their physician before the procedure.

FLAP DESIGN

There are 3 basic flap designs; 2 are traditional mainstays (Triangular, Ochsenbein-Luebke) and the third a variation of a periodontal surgical incision, the papilla-base flap.

The triangular flap design entails a full sulcular incision at least one tooth mesial and distal of the intended surgical field. The blade tip is in contact with the crest of alveolar bone throughout the incision, severing the periosteum, and carried through the sulcus and into each interdental papilla. As each papilla is incised, it can be gently reflected using the scalpel blade to ensure that a complete cut has been made. A vertical releasing incision is then made, originating at the line angle of the most anterior tooth of the flap, and drawn apically parallel to the long axis of the adjacent roots (**Fig. 1**).

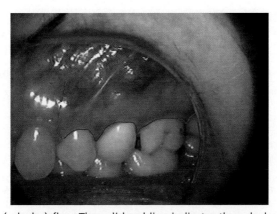

Fig. 1. Triangular (sulcular) flap. The solid red line indicates the sulcular incision from the mesial of tooth #12 to the distal of tooth #15; the dotted line represents the vertical releasing incision parallel to the root of tooth #11. Note the swelling in the mucobuccal fold near the MB apex of tooth #14.

The soft tissue of the flap is then reflected, starting in the vertical releasing incision and proceeding coronally/distally/apically, undermining and releasing the periosteum until full reflection is achieved and the surgical site is uncovered.

The Ochsenbein-Luebke flap was the design of choice in the maxillary anterior when there were concerns about exposure of crown margins or gingival recession following apical surgery (**Fig. 2**). This flap requires that the incision be contained within the attached gingiva, with at least 2 mm between the depth of the sulcus and the incision line. The band of attached gingiva should also be wide enough so that the incision line does not cross the mucogingival junction into the alveolar mucosa. It is imperative that the sulcus depths be mapped, and there are specific instruments made for this purpose called pocket markers, designed like college pliers, with one jaw configured like a periodontal probe and the other having a small "tooth" or projection on the tissue side of the jaw. These instruments are available in left- and right-side models to allow for correct orientation and adaptation to the tooth. The periodontal jaw is placed against the facial surface of the crown of each tooth, inserted to the depth of the facial sulcus at 3 points, and the handles are gently squeezed to bring the pointed end of the opposite jaw into contact with the facial gingival; this creates a series of bleeding points apical to each crown, representative of the depth of each individual sulcus. The incision is made 2 to 3 mm apical to these bleeding points, in a scalloped fashion to mimic the contour of the respective gingival crests. The incision is carried at least 1 to 2 teeth mesial and distal to the intended surgical site, with a vertical releasing incision terminating at both ends. The flap is reflected as with the triangular design, starting at one end of the incision and progressing to the opposite side. Although chosen to reduce the potential for exposed crown margins, this design is contraindicated in cases where a large apical lesion is present or there is an inadequate band of attached gingiva.[15–20]

The papilla-base flap could be best termed a hybrid variation of a full sulcular and split-thickness incisions, and has been suggested to prevent the gingival recession seen with the aforementioned 2 flap designs.[21] This flap consists of 2 vertical releasing incisions, connected by intrasulcular incisions in the cervical areas of the planned reflection concomitant with the papilla-based split-thickness variation. The split-thickness incision is accomplished in 2 steps: the first is a shallow cut, meant to sever the

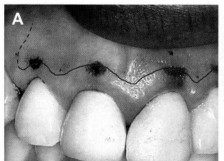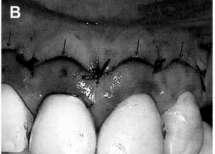

Fig. 2. (*A*) Ochsenbein-Luebke flap. The solid red line is the scalloped incision in the attached gingiva. The purple dots, made with a Gentian Violet stick, denote the probing depth plus 2 mm at the facial surface of each tooth in the proposed flap. The incision connects these dots together as one line, with vertical releasing incisions (*dotted lines*) at the terminal ends of the flap. (*B*) Ochsenbein-Luebke flap. The suturing of the coapted "points" of the flap correctly readapt the tissues. More sutures will be added to secure the flap (*arrows*).

epithelium and connective tissue to a depth of 1.5 mm from the surface of the gingiva, subscribing a curved line, perpendicular to the gingival margin, and connecting one side of the papilla to the other. The second cut is more vertical in nature, tracing the original incision but deep enough to contact the alveolar bone margin (**Fig. 3**). This cut will produce a split-thickness flap at the apical third of the base of the papilla.

This split-thickness incision is joined by the intrasulcular cut(s) at the cervical margin, completing the release of the marginal gingival complex. The intended flap is then reflected as a full-thickness mucoperiosteal event, apically positioned as dictated by the intended operative site. The one crucial caveat is the choice of scalpel blade; it should not exceed 2.5 mm in width, to allow for the delicate course of the incision and minimize inadvertent overcutting of the tissue. Although very predictable in terms of minimizing soft tissue recession, this is a very challenging flap design to execute and, if the tissues are mishandled, primary coaptation of the epithelial margins will be compromised; necrosis of the affected sections will occur and lead to formation of a surgical scar.[22] Also incumbent in this flap design is the size of the sutures used in closure; 7-0 to 8-0 polypropylene monofilament, at least 2 placed per papilla.

ERGONOMICS AND POSITIONING (PATIENT/SURGEON)

One of the most frustrating aspects of microscopic surgery is the correct positioning of the DOM relative to the patient and operative field. Indeed, a recent survey indicated almost 77% of those responding claimed some difficulty in access and visualization using the operating microscope.[23] Improper positional technique has long been recognized in the medical field, and guidelines to enhance performance and limit fatigue have been presented.[24,25] In endodontic surgery, the position of the patient is not as important as the position of the root apex and the immediate surgical field. This orientation forms the foundation on which the remainder of the microsurgical procedures is based. To begin, the patient is positioned in a supine to slightly Trende-lenberg attitude so that the surgical osteotomy site is most superior in the operating field. This position can vary from the patient simply turning their head to actually laying on their side. The patient can then be stabilized for comfort in this new position using rolled-up surgical towels, "donut" style headrests, or memory foam pillows. The

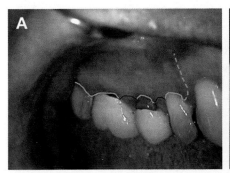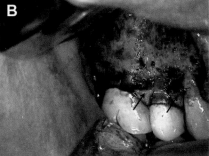

Fig. 3. (*A*) Papilla-based flap. The green lines denote the full sulcular portion of the incision around the cervical of each tooth, the red lines are the split-thickness incisions for the papillas involved, and the dotted green line is the vertical releasing incision. Note from the text that the papilla incisions are made with 2 different angles and depths. (*B*) Papilla-based flap reflection. The arrows point to the split-thickness reflection of each papilla. Note the long tissue bed of each papilla, especially between the 2 premolars.

surgeon then takes position at the head of the patient, the 11 to 12 O'clock orientation. The operator's chair height is adjusted so that the angle formed between the thigh and lower part of the foot is a minimum of 90°, and the spine is comfortably straight. The patient's chair is then raised or lowered so that the surgeon can maintain his or her elbows close to his body, passively bent at a neutral 90°. There are several companies that manufacture surgeon's chairs that have elbow rests incorporated into them, affording support of the forearms and elbows. Once positioned, the surgeon's arms and hands should not deviate from the core-centric position; this affords the greatest dexterity and precise micro-control, while limiting fatigue and strain trembling.[26,27] The microscope is last positioned with the line of sight axis perpendicular to the soft tissue field of the intended flap, and the binocular eyepieces adjusted to a comfortable height relative to the operator.

The selected flap design is then incised, the soft tissue reflected, and the retractor(s) stabilized on the cortical plate. The retractors must be in contact with the bone to avoid inadvertent impingement of the reflected soft tissue or other vital structures such as the mental nerve. The retractors must also be positioned at some distance from the surgical site to afford access for visualization and manipulation of the instruments. However, the extent of the reflection is not as broad as with other oral surgical procedures; rather, the reflection forms a narrow corridor bordered by the edges of the flap. This corridor not only minimizes the trauma to the soft tissues but desiccation of the cortical plate as well. This retraction can be augmented by the assistant using a second retraction instrument such as a Seldin or Pritchard style periosteal elevator to gently redirect a lip or section of the flap that has prolapsed into the field, especially during the osteotomy and root end resection phases of the procedure. Once retraction is complete and stable, the patient is readjusted so that the cortical plate/tooth long axis of the surgical site is parallel to the floor and most superior in the field (**Fig. 4**).

ERGONOMICS AND POSITIONING (PATIENT/SURGEON/DOM): SITE SPECIFIC

Although there is no one correct way to position the microscope relative to the field, an excellent guide would be to visualize what a direct line of sight to the field would be,

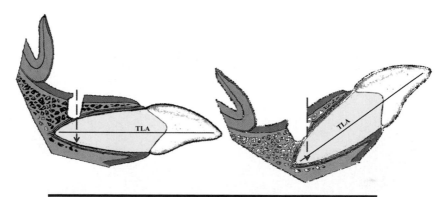

Floor

Fig. 4. The correct positioning (*left*) for the tooth long axis relative to the floor on the left. Positioning in this manner allows for the resection to be "gravity driven," dropping straight down toward the floor, making a right angle cut with regard to the facial-palatal direction. On the right, because the angle is incorrect, the osteotomy is larger and the resection is angled from facial to palatal.

then position the line of sight of the microscope along that imaginary line. Inclinable optics allow for the microscope to assume different vertical attitudes relative to 90°, and a shift of as little as 20° in either direction will enable the surgeon to look past the head of the handpiece to the end of a burr, or use direct vision to examine a resected root end. It is also imperative to have the microscope visual axis (MVA) parallel to the root long axis (RLA) at the selected resection level; if the observation position is skewed off-angle, the resection will mimic that angle (**Fig. 5**). This section explains the basics of positioning for the microscope; more details concerning the actual root end procedures follow in later sections. For the 4 major quadrants, the respective position guidelines are presented.

MAXILLARY ANTERIOR

The head of the microscope is tilted slightly off from direct vertical, angling from the crown of the tooth toward the apex (**Fig. 6**). This angle will alleviate the superimposition effect of the head of the handpiece; bring the tip of the selected burr into view. Decortication of the intended apical site, if not already exposed by pathologic fenestration, is affected by a small round bur (#2–4) or other specialized bone bur (Lindeman Bone Bur). Care should be taken not to unintentionally gouge the selected root surface during this discovery phase. Use of a nonaerosol producing handpiece, such as an

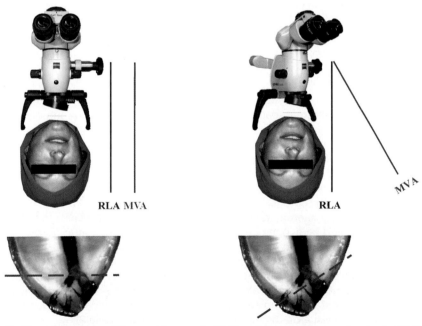

RLA MVA　　　　　　RLA　　　MVA

Fig. 5. The relationship of the root long axis (RLA) and the microscope visual axis (MVA). If the microscope and, by extension, the surgeon are positioned in the same line as the long axis of the root at the selected resection site, then the line of resection will be parallel to the surgeon's chest, an ergonomically reproducible path. This positioning will ensure the correct mesial-distal angulation. When a disparity exists, as shown on the right, the surgeon is guided by their body position and line of sight, not the position of the root tip, and an angled resection is made.

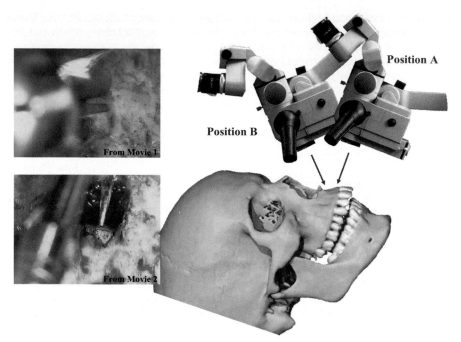

Fig. 6. The correct inclination of the microscope and patient for maxillary anterior surgery. Position A and Movie 1 are for the resection; position B and Movie 2 are for the inspection, root end preparation (REP), and root end filling (REF).

Impact Air (Palisades Dental, Englewood, NJ, USA) will reduce the amount of occult spray in the field and improve visibility without compromising cooling of the bur and bone. Following identification of the selected apex, the osteotomy is enlarged to enable curettage of any lesion present and isolate the root tip from the surrounding surgical crypt. How large an osteotomy should be is predicated on the native size of the lesion, adequate access for the armamentarium, and proximity to vital structure such as the mental nerve, mandibular canal, or maxillary sinus. In a phrase: it should be as small as possible but as large as practical.

Once the root tip is isolated, the surgeon and DOM are repositioned so that they are parallel to the long axis of the root at the selected level of the resection, *not the long axis of the tooth*, and the coronal-apical inclination is reestablished. With the direct line of sight to the bur tip restored, the root end is resected (Movie 1, available along with all other movies cited here in the on-line version of this article at: http://www.dental.theclinics.com). Once resection is complete, the microscope is then angled from apex to crown to allow for inspection of the resected root surface with direct vision (Movie 2). The angle will, of course, depend on the extent and quality of the retraction. Following the resection, the operator will be using micromirrors to more accurately assess the accuracy and completeness of the resected surface. This same angle will also be used to visualize the root end preparation (see Movie 2).

MANDIBULAR ANTERIOR

The positioning is relatively the same, with a few notable exceptions:

(a) Positioning of the cortical plate parallel to the floor may not be possible; this should be taken into account during the root end resection and preparation phases. In many instances, rather than recline the patient to an uncomfortable angle, it may be enough to have them elevate their chin slightly to affect this parallel position (**Fig. 7**) (Movies 3 and 4).

(b) The second angle, coming from the apex to the crown, again may be compromised by the limitations of the reflection and the angle of the patient, but the solution may again be as simple as having the patient elevate the chin for a short period of time to enable the correct line of sight.

MAXILLARY AND MANDIBULAR POSTERIOR

The limiting factor here is the ability of the patient to present the cortical plate parallel to the floor. Using rolled surgical towels or pillows to prop the back of the patient will allow them to comfortably lie on their side in the dental chair, affording a more favorable attitude to the surgical site. An anesthesiologist's "donut" or small pillow can also be placed under the patient's head to gently cushion it in this new position. Failure to achieve this presentation of the surgical field often results in a misdirected "tunneling" of the osteotomy, with the potential for inadvertently damaging adjacent roots or structures (**Fig. 8**). Also, retraction in the most posterior of sites is inhibited by the xygoma or external oblique ridge, and may require repositioning of the retractor(s). Otherwise, the previous rules of positioning of the microscope hold true with respect to the osteotomy, root end resection/inspection, and preparation (**Figs. 9** and **10**) (Movies 5–8).

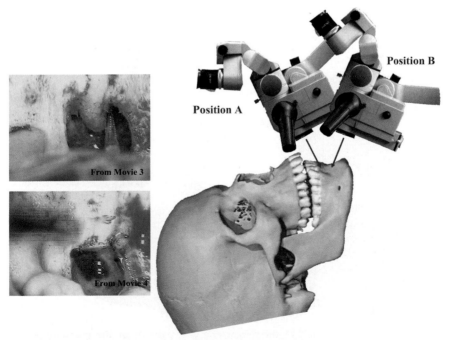

Fig. 7. The correct inclination of the microscope and patient for the mandibular anterior surgery. Position A and Movie 3 are for the resection; position B and Movie 4 are for the inspection, REP, and REF.

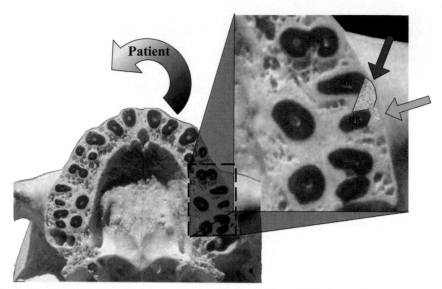

Fig. 8. The magnified area of root apices teeth #13, #14, and #15 shows the correct osteotomy approach (*green arrow*) for the distobuccal root of tooth #14. However, if the patient is facing straight forward, the field of view is distorted at higher magnification, and the approach angle is often too far mesial, resulting in a grazing or gouging of the MB root (*red arrow*). Turning the patient so that the cortical plate of the site is superior in the field alleviates this difficulty.

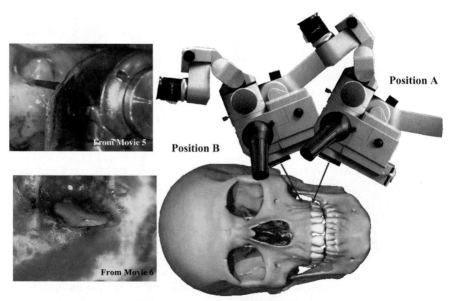

Fig. 9. The correct inclination of the microscope and patient for the maxillary posterior surgery. Position A and Movie 5 are for the resection; position B and Movie 6 are for the inspection, REP, and REF. Note the bow-tie effect on the resected root surface of this MB root.

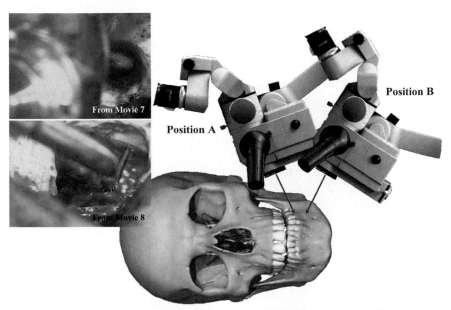

Fig. 10. The correct inclination of the microscope and patient for the mandibular posterior surgery. Position A and Movie 7 are for the resection; position B and Movie 8 are for the inspection, REP, and REF. Note the harvesting of the root apex after resection, and the 2 canals it demonstrates (one filled, one uninstrumentcd/filled).

ROOT END RESECTION

This phase is perhaps the most pivotal of the surgical procedure, as errors here are magnified with respect to the subsequent root end preparation and successful sealing of the apical extent of the root canal system. The carpenters' axiom of "measure twice, cut once" has great significance, as root structure cannot be replaced once it has been removed, so careful consideration must be given to the length and angle of the resection process.

LENGTH

First and foremost are the restorative implications of the resection with regard to crown-root ratio. There are histologic guidelines for how much of the root end should be removed but if, in doing so, the integrity and stability of the remaining tooth is compromised, alternative treatment options should be explored. If there is sufficient root length in sound bone, then the amount of root apex that is removed is dictated by the prevalence and distribution of the apical ramifications the surgeon hopes to eliminate. As the accompanying diagram shows (**Fig. 11**), a resection level of 3 mm from the anatomic apex will eliminate 93% of lateral canals and 98% of any other ramifications such as deltas, fins, and so forth.[28] Coupled with a root end preparation depth of 3 mm, 6 mm of infectious etiology in the canal space will have been effectively treated. There are, however, 2 notable exceptions to this rule. First, if the level of resection is such that it leaves a root geometry that is significantly curved at that level, then the root end preparation will be compromised (**Fig. 12**). The preparation tips, by design, are 3 mm long, and are not designed to follow curves like a root canal file.

	1 millimeter	2 millimeters	3 millimeters
Apical Ramifications	52%	78%	98%
Lateral canals	40%	86%	93%

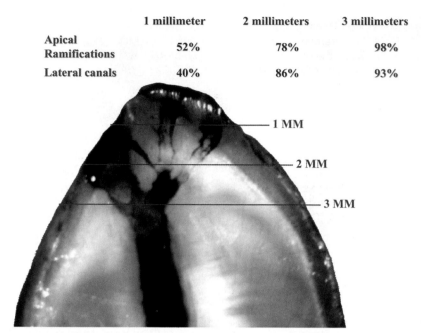

Fig. 11. The relationship of resection level and canal ramifications eliminated in this canine apex. (*Data from* Kim S, Kratchman S. Modern endodontic surgery concepts and practice: a review. J Endod 2006;32:601–23.)

Hence, the preparation will be shallower than required because of the tip's impact on the curve or, if forced longer, can in fact perforate the external root surface. This situation can be remedied by increasing the length of the resection past the curve, provided the overall length of the remaining portion of the root does not compromise the crown-root ratio.

The other exception occurs when the root in question has undergone a resorptive process, and is shorter than normal. In this instance, part of that ideal 3-mm length

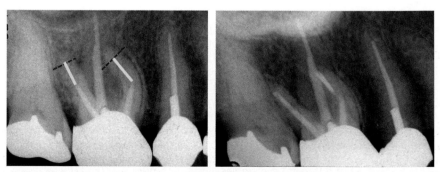

Fig. 12. The preoperative radiograph of tooth #3 demonstrates the dissimilar curves of the roots, and the correspondingly different angles of resection for each root apex. Note that the resection of the MB apex is slightly shorter so as not to impact the REP into the curve. The postoperative radiograph shows the REF to be well centered and to the correct depth.

has been eliminated involuntarily. Comparison of the root length of the contralateral tooth can assist in determining how much more of the apex needs to be removed, if any. At the very least, the resorbed root apex would likely need to be flattened somewhat to allow for efficient root end preparation and filling/finishing.

ANGLE

Before the introduction of the microscope, resected root ends were routinely beveled to enable the surgeon to visualize the resected surface(s). It was not uncommon for bevels of 30°, 45°, or even greater to be placed because of "convenience." This beveling was most often rendered by with a #4 to #6 round burr attached to a large, straight nose cone handpiece, such as a Stryker, or with a fissure burr in a conventional slow-speed handpiece. This severe angle contributed to gross apical leakage and often failure of the apical surgery. In 1989, Tidmarsh and Arrowsmith[29] examined the implications of the beveled resection (45°–60°) with regard to dentinal tubule concentration in young and old teeth, and the depth of the effective retrograde seal. These investigators concluded that the potential for leakage was greatest when the bevel was steep and the retrograde filling did not extend deeper than the coronal aspect of the beveled surface. This concept was elaborated upon with the work of Gilheany and colleagues 1994.[30] Twenty-seven single-rooted teeth were selected and their root apices were resected at 0°, 30°, and 45°. Apical preparations were created and sequentially filled with a glass ionomer (Ketac Silver). The apical microleakage and dentin permeability were measured by observing and quantifying the fluid flow in a hydraulic conductance apparatus as described by Derkson and colleagues in 1986.[31] Gilheaney and colleagues concluded that: (1) the amount of leakage increased as the slope of the bevel increased; (2) increasing the depth of the retrograde filling decreased the microleakage; and (3) optimum/minimum depths for the retrogrades were as follows: 0° = 1 mm, 30° = 2.1 mm, 45° = 2.5 mm (**Fig. 13**).

Bur selection for the root apex removal is almost a matter of personal choice. However, here are some guidelines based on the literature[32–34]:

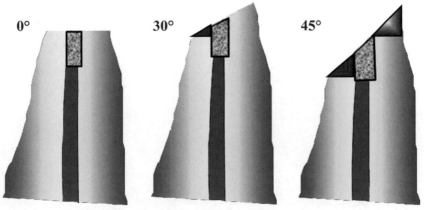

Fig. 13. The impact of different bevel angles, and the amount of lateral leakage through the exposed dentinal tubules to the REF (*blue triangles*). The red triangle in the 45° bevel would represent contaminated tubules left after such a resection in an infected root apex. (*Data from* Gilheany PA, Figdor D, Tyas MJ. Apical dentin permeability and microleakage associated with root end resection and retrograde filling. J Endod 1994;20:22–6.)

(a) Straight or tapered carbide fissure configuration, long enough to span the depth of the apex, is advised. If a tapered fissure is chosen, the angle created by the taper should be taken into account during the resection to maintain as close of a 0° bevel as possible.

(b) Avoid coarse diamond or crosscut fissure configurations as these create surface roughness and irregularities, making it difficult to finish the REF properly.

(c) Use of the bur in a high-speed handpiece with copious coolant is advised. It is also recommended that this coolant stream not be air driven, as this could potentially induce an air embolism effect in the soft tissues of the surgical field. An example of such a handpiece is the Impact Air, available with or without fiber optic capability.

The technique of the resection is not the "chainsaw" cutting of a tree trunk, but rather akin to the slicing of a piece of bread. In the former action, the coolant would fail to effectively reach the interface of the bur and tooth surface being cut, allowing for the dentinal surface to become overheated and burned. By using the tip of the bur and making progressively deeper passes across the root tip surface, not only will the coolant flush and cool the resection cut but also the first few passes will create a "guide slot" in the root. If any adjustments to length or angle are required, they are easily corrected at this time without undue, and irreversible, damage to the root. This guide slot also serves as a "pilot reference" to maintain the correct angle throughout the resection. Some operators prefer to shave the root end rather than resect it. The author feels that this has the potential to cloud the issue of how much has really been removed, and the shaving of an infected root end disperses just that much more pathogenic material into the surrounding crypt.

Once the apex (ices) has been removed, the first observation made should be of the resected tip cut surface (**Fig. 14**). This view will very often mirror the cut surface of the remaining root, offering a preview of what the surgeon is to expect in terms of number of canals, filled or unfilled, isthmuses, fractures, and so forth. Such observations can also reveal the smoothness of the cut, and whether the resection was complete; a jagged edge along the perimeter of the root usually indicates that portion of the root being broken off, rather than cut cleanly. The situation is confirmed clinically by examining the remaining root surface, either directly or in a micromirror.

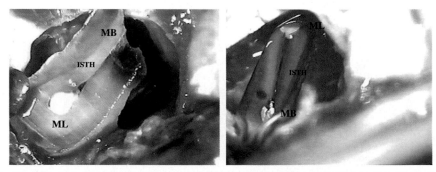

Fig. 14. The picture on the left shows a root tip harvested after resection in this surgical re-treatment. The black stain near the MB canal is from the amalgam retrograde. Note the long isthmus seen in this tip; it is the mirror image of what can be expected when the resected surface of the root is viewed. The picture on the right is the micromirror view of the resected surface; an exact replica of the observation made from the harvested root tip.

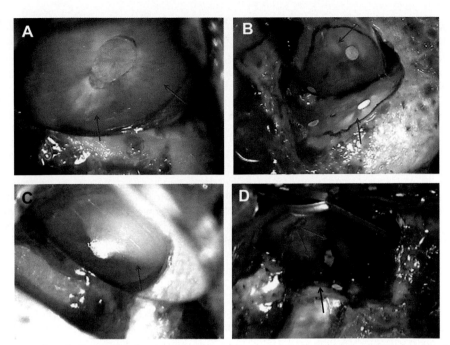

Fig. 15. (*A, B*) The radial dentin pattern in an anterior and posterior tooth, respectively. (*C, D*) The bow-tie effect. (*C*) The dentinal tubules of the transitional lines as they appear naturally; (*D*) the tubules stained at the transitional line angles from a coronally leaking obturation.

The remainder of the crypt is curetted to remove any remnants of soft tissue, sufficient hemostasis is either maintained or attained (explained in the following section), and the resected root end is disclosed with methylene blue, caries indicator, or other nontoxic dye. Subsequent observations of the root end(s) with a micromirror are made to assess the conditions of the site: are there incomplete resections, indicated by an irregular periodontal ligament perimeter or "dog-eared" projection of dentin? Are there extra roots/ canals present, evident by the staining or lack of it? Are there fractures or isthmuses, and what is their location and extent? All of these points need to be cataloged and resolved before any root end preparation. One interesting observation can be made without the aid of any disclosing solution. The author terms this the "Bow-Tie" effect, and it is readily evident on the wet, resected surface of the root (**Fig. 15**). These faint lines are not fractures, but represent the transitional line angles of the root dentin/tubules. Because the dentinal tubules refract light differently, depending on their orientation to the light source, they will present a different appearance when viewed with incident

---

Box 1
Water prism fluid effect

Movie 9 shows the prism effect of a clear fluid in the crypt of tooth #24. With the proper fluid level, it is possible to view the resected surface without the micromirror. Without altering the position of the DOM, the fluid is removed to reveal how much of the light and view was being "bent" by the prism effect of the fluid.

> **Box 2**
> **Ferric sulfate hemostasis technique**
> Movie 10. Placement of a pellet moistened with ferric sulfate into this grossly bleeding crypt. Note the immediate blackening of the occult blood and pellet. The end of the video shows a curette creating a fresh bleeding surface, and sloughing of the necrotized tissue.

light. This appearance is the apical manifestation of what the author has termed "radial dentin" seen in the coronal chambers of dystrophically obliterated teeth.[35] This "radial dentin" tracks back to the obliterated pulp space, serving as a map to the narrowed canal. The radial dentin, apically, will point to the central location of the canal space and isthmus. This indication is especially important if the dye used did not disclose any canal/isthmus but the radial dentin suggests that it is present; the conclusion must then be drawn that the resection level did not cut through, and thereby expose, the canal/isthmus enough to capture the dye. The clinical decision is then made to either root end prepare according to the radial dentin outlines, or resect slightly more of the root end to reveal the suspected space(s).

One last observation "trick" involves the principle of a prism and its ability to bend light. This "water prism" is especially useful in the mandibular anterior apices, where space in the crypt is often cramped and bleeding slightly. After resection, the crypt is rinsed with sterile saline until it runs clear but, rather than suction the site dry, the saline is allowed to remain in the crypt. The level of the fluid can be adjusted through judicious suctioning with a microcannula, until the whole root end surface can be observed. Not only will this facilitate the accurate positioning of the USREP (UltraSonic Root End Preparation) tip without a micromirror, but the fluid itself offers a weak hemostatic tamponade effect (Movie 9; for movie description, see **Box 1**).

HEMOSTASIS

Before the USREP, the absolute hemostasis of the crypt needs to be achieved. Although the best hemostasis is achieved preoperatively with the anesthetic, a prolonged surgery or systemic conditions may tax the effectiveness of the Lidocaine 1:50,000. Most agents effect hemostasis by either by direct heme-agglutination or by triggering the natural clotting cascade of the patient. Of the two, the natural effect is preferable because it lasts for a relatively longer period of time. These agents, and their mode of action, are as follows.

Heme-Agglutination

Solutions
Ferric sulfate or ferric subsulfate is the generic name for this agent. Depending on the concentration of the chemical, it is also known by the trade names: Astringedent (Ultradent Products Inc, UT, USA) Viscostat, Stasis (Cut-Trol Ichthys Enterprises, Mobile, AL, USA), and Monsel's.

> **Box 3**
> **Hemodette hemostasis technique**
> Movie 11. Placement of a blue Hemodette pellet and hemostasis after 3 minutes.

Box 4
ActCel hemostasis technique

Movie 12. Placement of the material at the mesiobuccal (MB) apex of tooth #19. Demonstrates the material turning to a jelly, and the excess is removed. After hemostasis is achieved, the crypt is rinsed and the REF is placed.

The most efficient delivery is via small microbrushes dipped into a dappen dish containing the solution, and then the moist tips are discretely applied to any small bleeding points. The agglutinated proteins coagulate and form a physical plug almost immediately, and hemostasis is preserved so long as this plug remains undisturbed. Although extremely effective, all remnants of the ferric sulfate must be removed, and a fresh bleeding surface reestablished (Movie 10; for movie description, see **Box 2**). Otherwise, significant and adverse effects on the osseous and soft tissue healing of the site can be expected.[36,37] The necrotizing effects, along with the difficulty in controlling the distribution and complete elimination of this agent, strongly preclude its selection in areas of neurovascular concern, namely, mandibular nerve, mental foramen, maxillary sinus, and floor of the nose.

Gels

Hemodette (20% buffered aluminum chloride gel, DUX Dental, Oxnard, CA, USA) is a water-soluble agent with agglutination properties similar to ferric sulfate, but without the deleterious side effects. This agent is packaged as 2 impregnated cotton pellets with an excess of gel in a sterile container resembling a prophy cup. Delivery is with the cotton pellet or, using a microbrush, painting the crypt with the free gel. In addition to the heme-agglutination effect, the gel itself forms a sort of passive barrier to any minor bleeder. The blue color makes it readily identifiable in the site, and it is easily rinsed from the crypt with saline at the conclusion of the procedure (Movie 11; for movie description, see **Box 3**).

There are other gauze-based products such as ActCel (ActSys, Westlake Village, CA, USA), HemCon (HemCon Medical Technologies, Portland, OR, USA), and Blood-Stop (LifeSciencePlus, Palo Alto, CA, USA) that, when moistened with saline or blood from the site, break down into a gel matrix, exerting the same combination of mild tamponade and heme-agglutination as the Hemodette, and that are just as easily removed. (Movie 12; for movie description, see **Box 4**).

Physiologic Clotting Agents

These products are, by and large, either bovine or porcine derived connective tissue matrices that initiate the patient's own clotting cascade at the site. The advantage of this type of hemostasis is that it is usually longer lasting and more predictable in effect. Although Avitene (Avitene microfibrillar collagen hemostat, Davol Inc, Warwick, RI, USA) is the most effective and well known of this category, it is difficult to place and expensive (Movie 13; for movie description, see **Box 5**). A reasonable substitute would

---

Box 5
Avitene hemostasis technique

Movie 13. Placement of the microfibrillar type, and the exceptional hemostasis after 2 minutes in situ.

Box 6
Colla Plug hemostasis technique

Movie 14. Placement of a small Colla Plug disc shows adequate hemostasis after 2 minutes.

be either CollaPlug or CollaTape (Zimmer Dental, Carlsbad, CA, USA). The tape dressing can be easily cut to fit the osteotomy, and the plug can be sliced into small discs and placed over the bleeding sites. Gentle tamponade will accelerate the effect, although once the material is removed, the clotting effect will deteriorate within a few minutes (Movie 14; for movie description, see **Box 6**).

ROOT END PREPARATION

Since their introduction by Carr in the early 1990s, the use of the USREP tip has refined the technique and practice of this phase of the surgery. USREP tips have evolved from smooth stainless steel tips of limited configurations to a myriad of multiple bends and angles, with coatings of diamond or zirconium nitride (**Fig. 16**). The safety, efficiency, and directions for use have been well investigated in the literature, and are considered the standard for root end preparations.[38–42] There are several manufacturers of these

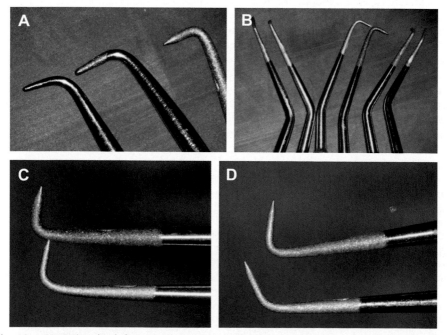

Fig. 16. USREP tips. (*A, left to right*) A stainless steel tip, a diamond-coated tip, and a zirconium nitride (ZN)-coated tip. (*B*) the assorted tip configurations for the ZN (ProUltraSurgical tips, Dentsply-Tulsa Dental, Tulsa, OK, USA). (*C*) The tip diameter of the smaller #1 universal tip, and the larger #2 universal tip. (*D*) The different tip angles of the #3 and #4 posterior surgical tips. These different angles can accommodate different surgical presentation angles of the root end without having to affect awkward handpiece positions.

Box 7
USREP tip guide

Movie 15. A reference notch is made on the cortical plate of tooth #14 MB root with the side of the US tip. This notch, made parallel to the long axis of the root at the resection site, serves as a visual reference during root end preparation to maintain the proper angle of the USREP tip.

---

specialized tips, and most are interchangeable with regard to the attachment to a generating unit.

TECHNIQUE

Although the universal tips are designed for anterior teeth, and tri-angled tips for posterior locations, there is no rule as to where a particular tip can or cannot be used; the determining factor is access with the selected tip attached, and visibility during its use. In single canal roots, the tip is placed into the center of the gutta percha, if present, or the center of the canal space. The tip is energized, with enough coolant delivered through the tip to cool and flush the preparation site. The tip is allowed to passively seek its way down the canal, and this will happen readily if gutta percha is in the canal. Any high-pitched squeal from the tip indicates either binding in a small, uninstrumented canal, or that the tip is traversing off-angle. Visual inspection with a micromirror is prudent at this point to ensure that the preparation is remaining centered in the canal. A groove in the buccal cortical plate, placed with the side of the USREP tip, and parallel to the long axis of the root, will also aid in the correct angulation of the preparation, especially at higher magnifications (Movie 15; for movie description, see **Box 7**). The preparation is complete when the full depth of the tip is reached, usually 3 mm. In a root with multiple canals and an isthmus joining them (ie, the MB root of the maxillary first molar), the 2 canals (MB1 and MB2) are prepared separately to establish the correct angulation of the preparation, then the isthmus connecting them is prepped at the same angle (Movie 16; for movie description, see **Box 8**). This action can be performed either directly or after tracing a small groove in the isthmus with the USREP tip dry. This latter procedure creates a trough that will be easier to replicate once the tip is activated with coolant streaming into the site, but caution should be exercised not to overheat the tip or the root end by prolonged dry cutting. These coated tips are most efficient when they are new; for that reason, it is the author's opinion that they should be considered a single-use item.

The identification and preparation of the isthmus is crucial to the sealing, and subsequent successful healing, of the root end. Although some have designated 5 or 6 types of isthmuses, they are actually permutations, based on the level of resection in a particular root, of 2 basic types: partial and complete. First identified as a prominent surgical

---

Box 8
USREP technique

Movie 16 shows the preparation, using a new USREP tip, of the MB root of tooth #3. The MB1 and MB2 canals are prepared first, then the isthmus is prepared maintaining the identical angle between the 2 main canals. The preparation is viewed at completion in the micromirror.

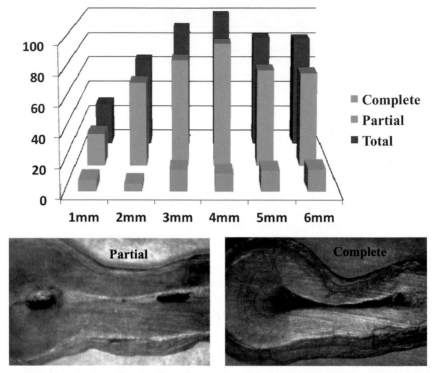

Fig. 17. In the MB root of a maxillary first molar with 2 canals, the table demonstrates an isthmus at the ideal resection length (3–4 mm) 100% of the time. (*Data from* Weller RN, Niemczyk SP, Kim S. Incidence and position of the canal isthmus. Part 1. Mesiobuccal root of the maxillary first molar. J Endod 1995;21:380–3.)

consideration in the MB root of a maxillary first molar (**Fig. 17**),[43] it has evolved to include any root that has the potential to contain 2 or more canals,[44,45] and should be considered present until judged otherwise.

ROOT END FILLING

Although every restorative material has been used, at one time or another, as a REF, selection of today's REF is predicated on whether it is contained within a root end preparation (REP) or not. For situations whereby a REP can be created, the material of choice is Mineral Trioxide Aggregate (MTA) (ProRoot MTA, Dentsply-Tulsa Dental, Tulsa, OK, USA). This compound is easy to mix, not cumbersome to place, and extremely biocompatible.[46–53] MTA is manufactured in white and gray formulations virtually identical in composition. The only caveat is that the material must be placed

---

Box 9
MAPS root end filling technique

Movie 17. Placement of MTA using a MAPS syringe. MTA is overfilled, the excess compacted with the back of a Molt curette, and the surface of the MTA dried and wiped to contour with a microbrush. Micromirror view shows 2 canals in this buccal root of tooth #12.

> **Box 10**
> **MTA air-dry technique**
>
> Movie 18. The soft excess MTA is dried with an indirect airstream from the Stropko Irrigator tip. Once dried, the MTA is condensed with a ball burnisher and the excess is removed with a microbrush. The crypt is flushed with saline, and examined with a micromirror.

in a dry prep; excessive bleeding or moisture will wash the material away before setting. The most effective method to dry the REP is with a microtip attached to a Stropko Irrigator (J Bar B Co, Carefree, AZ, USA) syringe attachment. This device replaces the disposable tip of the triplex syringe, and the luer-lock end permits any size luer-lock needle tip or cannula to be readily attached. With the air pressure reduced to 3 to 5 psi, this device can direct a concentrated stream of air or water to the REP, either rinsing or drying it.

Placement of the MTA can be accomplished with a variety of instruments, from an inexpensive wipe-on block (Lee Endo Bloc, San Francisco, CA, USA) to a more sophisticated and costly syringe system (MAPS Roydent, Johnson City, TN, USA). (Movie 17; for movie description, see **Box 9**). Once the MTA is placed, a gentle steam of air from the Stropko is directed across the top of the REF to desiccate, and thereby firm or "skin" the exposed surface of the material, After 20 to 30 seconds, the surface of the REF is firm enough to carve and any excess can be gently wiped away with a microbrush (Movie 18; for movie description, see **Box 10**). The crypt may even be rinsed gently, provided the irrigant stream is not directed at the REF.

In instances whereby the depth of a post precludes a normal REP, then a bonded restoration such as Geristore (DenMat, Santa Maria, CA, USA) may be placed to seal the root end. The technique of using bonded restorations on unprepared root ends was introduced by Rud and colleagues,[54–57] and has enjoyed a great measure of success. However, as with the MTA, it is technique sensitive with respect to moisture, and the osteotomy is often enlarged to create a "high and dry" exposure of the

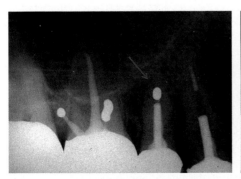
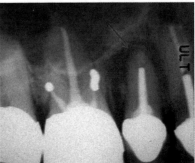

| Pre-operative | Post-operative |

Fig. 18. Preoperative radiograph of tooth #4 reveals a post placed nearly to the root apex, and a failing retrograde in place (*arrow*). A bonded restoration (Geristore) replaces the amalgam and is the REF of choice when a REP of conventional depth cannot be achieved. The postoperative radiograph reveals the faint radio-opacity of the REF, and the conventional surgery and REF on tooth #5.

Box 11
Geristore root end filling technique

Movie 19. Placement of Geristore in the apex of tooth #4. Note the close proximity of the post to the restoration.

---

root end. After saucering the root end, it is isolated, etched, and primed. The Geristore is a dual-cure material, so an orange filter should be placed between the DOM light source and the surgical site to prevent premature curing of the material. The REF is either troweled or syringed onto the root end, the filter removed, and the material cured with the appropriate light source, then contoured to the root outline (**Fig. 18**) (Movie 19; for movie description, see **Box 11**).

SUTURING/CLOSURE

After the site has been cleansed of all debris, the underside of the flap(s) is gently rinsed with sterile saline and coapted back to the original positions. A moistened gauze is placed over the coapted tissue, and gentle pressure is applied for approximately 5 minutes. This procedure effectively expresses any occult blood under the flap, and initiates a preliminary attachment of the tissues. The flap is secured with either interrupted or sling sutures; the choice of type and size is dictated by the flap design and retention requirements. Postoperative instructions should include diet and hygiene restrictions, pain medication guidelines and, most importantly, chilling of the overlying facial surface with ice (preferably in a zip-lock bag wrapped with a moist washcloth). The application of cold controls the amount of swelling from the rebound vasodilatation phase, and therefore reduces the postoperative potential for discomfort from swelling. Chilling should continue for the first 24 hours postoperatively (10–15 minutes on, 5 minutes off) except while sleeping. Suture removal, in uncomplicated cases, is normally 1 to 3 days after the operation.

SUMMARY

Today, endodontic surgeons are able to render a level of service with confidence and great precision that 20 years ago would have seemed unattainable by any standard. The development of a sophisticated armamentarium, groundbreaking techniques, and the willingness to embrace them is the future of the specialty. The next 20 years should eclipse anything previously dreamt of, if the last 20 are any barometer of things to come.

REFERENCES

1. Shelton M. Working in a very small place; the making of a neurosurgeon. New York: W.W. Norton & Company; 1989. p. 91–3.
2. Selden HS. The role of the dental operating microscope in endodontics. Pa Dent J 1986;53:36.
3. Selden HS. The role of the dental operating microscope in improved nonsurgical treatment of "calcified" canals. Oral Surg Oral Med Oral Pathol 1989;68:93.
4. Selden HS. The dental operating microscope and its slow acceptance. J Endod 2002;28:206.
5. Pecora G, Andreana S. Use of dental operating microscope in endodontic surgery. Oral Surg Oral Med Oral Pathol 1993;75(6):751.
6. Carr GB. Microscopes in endodontics. J Calif Dent Assoc 1992;20:55.

7. Mines P, Loushine R, WQest L, et al. Use of the microscope in endodontics: a report based on a questionnaire. J Endod 1999;25:755.
8. Kersten DD, Mines P, Sweet M. Use of the microscope in endodontics: results of a questionnaire. J Endod 2008;34:804.
9. Hargreaves KM, Khan A. Surgical preparation: anesthesia and hemostasis. Endodontic Topics 2005;11:32–55.
10. Gordon SM, Dionne RA, Brahim J, et al. Blockade of peripheral neuronal barrage reduces postoperative pain. Pain 1997;70:209.
11. Jackson DL, Moore PA, Hargreaves KM. Pre-operative non-steroidal anti-inflammatory medication for the prevention of postoperative dental pain. J Am Dent Assoc 1989;119:641.
12. Dionne RA. Suppresion of dental pain by the preoperative administration of flurbiprofen. Am J Med 1986;80:41.
13. Gutmann JL. Parameters of achieving quality anesthesia and hemostasis in surgical endodontics [review]. Anesth Pain Control Dent 1993;2:223.
14. Kim S, Retham S. Hemostasis in endodontic microsurgery. Dent Clin North Am 1997;41:499–513.
15. Johnson BR, Witherspoon DE. Periradicular surgery. In: Cohen, Hargreaves, editors. Pathways of the pulp. 9th edition. St. Louis (MO): Mosby; 2006. p. 744–5.
16. Pitt Ford Thomas R. Surgical treatment of apical periodontitis. In: Orstavik, Pitt Ford, editors. Essential endodontology. London: Blackwell Science Ltd; 1998. p. 282–3.
17. Arens DE. Practical lessons in endodontic surgery, Part I, lessons 1–7. Illinois: Quintessence Publishing Company; 1998.
18. Arens DE, Adams WR, DeCastro RA. Endodontic surgery, Chapter 1: considerations and indications for endodontic surgery. Philadelphia: Harper & Row; 1981. p. 1–13.
19. Gutman J, Harrison J. Surgical endodontics. St Louis (MO): Ishiyaku EuroAmerica, Inc; 1994. Chapter 6. p. 154–61.
20. Gutmann JL, Harrison JW. Posterior endodontic surgery: anatomical considerations and clinical techniques. Int Endod J 1985;18:8.
21. Velvart P. Papilla base incision: a new approach to recession-free healing of the interdental papilla after endodontic surgery. Int Endod J 2002;35:453–60.
22. Velvart P, Peters CI, Peters OA. Soft tissue management: suturing and wound closure. In: Trope M, editor, Endodontic topics, vol. 11. Copenhagen V (Denmark): Blackwell Munksgaard; 2005. p. 179–95.
23. Creasy JE, Mines P, Sweet M. Surgical trends among endodontists: the results of a web-based survey. J Endod 2009;35:30.
24. Berguer R. Surgery and ergonomics. Arch Surg 1999;134:1011.
25. Buffington CW, MacMurdo SD, Ryan CM. Body position affects manual dexterity. Anesth Analg 2006;102:1879.
26. Comes C, Valceanu A, Rusu D, et al. A study on the ergonomical working modalities using the dental operating microscope (DOM). Part 1: ergonomic principles in dental medicine. TMJ 2008;58(3–4):218.
27. Golenberg L, Cao A, Ellis RD, et al. Hand position effects on precision and speed in telerobotic surgery. Int J Med Robot 2007;3(3):217–23.
28. Kim S, Kratchman S. Modern endodontic surgery concepts and practice: a review. J Endod 2006;32:601–23.
29. Tidmarsh BG, Arrowsmith MG. Dentinal tubules at the root ends of apicected teeth: a scanning electron microscopic study. Int Endod J 1989;22:184–9.
30. Gilheany PA, Figdor D, Tyas MJ. Apical dentin permeability and microleakage associated with root end resection and retrograde filling. J Endod 1994;20:22–6.

31. Derkson GD, Pashley DH, Derkson ME. Microleakage measurement of selected restorative materials: a new in vitro method. J Prosthet Dent 1986; 56:435–40.
32. Gutmann JL. Perspectives on root-end resection. J Hist Dent 1999;47(3):135–6.
33. Morgan LA, Marshall JG. The topography of root ends resected with fissure burs and refined with two types of finishing burs. Oral Surg Oral Med Oral Pathol Oral Radiol Endod 1998;85:585.
34. Weston GD, Moule AJ, Bartold PM. A comparison in vitro of fibroblast attachment to resected root ends. Int Endod J 1999;32:444.
35. Niemczyk SP. Seeing is believeing: the impact of the operating microscope on nonsurgical endodontic treatment. Pract Proced Aesthet Dent 2003;15:395–9.
36. Lemon RR, Steel PJ, Jeansonne BG. Ferric sulfate hemostasis: effect on osseous wound healing. I. Left *in situ* for maximum exposure. J Endod 1993;19:170.
37. Jeansonne BG, Lemon RR, Boggs WS. Ferric sulfate hemostasis: effect on osseous wound healing. II. With curettage and irrigation. J Endod 1993;19: 174.
38. Gray GJ, Hatton JF, Holtzman DJ, et al. Quality of root-end preparations using ultrasonic and rotary instrumentation in cadavers. J Endod 2000;26:281.
39. Peters CI, Peters OA, Barbakow F. An in vitro study comparing root-end cavities prepared by diamond-coated and stainless steel ultrasonic retrotips. Int Endod J 2001;34:142.
40. Taschieri S, Testori T, Francetti L, et al. Effects of ultrasonic root end preparation on resected root surfaces: SEM evaluation. Oral Surg Oral Med Oral Pathol Oral Radiol Endod 2004;98(5):611–8.
41. De Bruyne MA, De Moor RJ. SEM analysis of the integrity of resected root apices of cadaver and extracted teeth after ultrasonic root-end preparation at different intensities. Int Endod J 2005;38:310.
42. Roy R, Chandler NP, Lin J. Peripheral dentin thickness after root-end cavity preparation. Oral Surg Oral Med Oral Pathol Oral Radiol Endod 2008;105(2): 263–6.
43. Weller RN, Niemczyk SP, Kim S. Incidence and position of the canal isthmus. Part 1. Mesiobuccal root of the maxillary first molar. J Endod 1995;21:380–3.
44. Von Arx T. Frequency and type of canal isthmuses in first molars detected by endoscopic inspection during periradicular surgery. Int Endod J 2005;38:160.
45. Mannocci F, Peru M, Sherriff M, et al. The isthmuses of the mesial root of mandibular molars: a micro-computed tomographic study. Int Endod J 2005;38:558.
46. Torabinejad M, Pitt Ford TR, McKendry DJ, et al. Histologic assessment of mineral trioxide aggregate as a root-end filling in monkeys. J Endod 1997;23:225.
47. Chong BS, Pitt Ford TR, Hudson MB. A prospective clinical study of mineral trioxide aggregate and IRM when used as root-end filling materials in endodontic surgery. Int Endod J 2003;36(8):520–6.
48. Bernabé PF, Gomes-Filho JE, Rocha WC, et al. Histological evaluation of MTA as a root-end filling material. Int Endod J 2007;40(10):758–65.
49. Holland R, de Souza V, Nery J, et al. Reaction of dogs' teeth to root canal filling with Mineral Trioxide Aggregate or a Glass Ionomer sealer. J Endod 1999;25:728.
50. Lindeboom JA, Frenken JW, Kroon FH, et al. A comparative prospective randomized clinical study of MTA and IRM as root-end filling materials in single-rooted teeth in endodontic surgery. Oral Surg Oral Med Oral Pathol Oral Radiol Endod 2005;100(4):495–500.
51. Saunders WP. A prospective clinical study of periradicular surgery using mineral trioxide aggregate as a root-end filling. J Endod 2008;34(6):660–5.

52. Camilleri J, Montesin FE, Papaioannou S, et al. Biocompatibility of two commercial forms of mineral trioxide aggregate. Int Endod J 2004;37:699.
53. Tanomaru-Filho M, Luis MR, Leonardo MR, et al. Evaluation of periapical repair following retrograde filling with different root-end filling materials in dog teeth with periapical lesions. Oral Surg Oral Med Oral Pathol Oral Radiol Endod 2006;102(1):127–32.
54. Rud J, Munksgaard EC, Andreasen JO, et al. Retrograde root filling with composite and a dentin-bonding agent. 1. Endod Dent Traumatol 1991;7:118.
55. Rud J, Munksgaard EC, Andreasen JO, et al. Retrograde root filling with composite and a dentin-bonding agent. 2. Endod Dent Traumatol 1991;7:126.
56. Rud J, Rud V, Munksgaard EC. Long term evaluation of root filling with dentin-bonded resin composite. J Endod 1996;22:90.
57. Rud J, Rud V, Munksgaard EC. Periapical healing of mandibular molars after root-end sealing with dentine-bonded composite. Int Endod J 2001;34:285.

Endodontic and Implant Algorithms

W.R. Bowles, DDS, MS, PhD[a],*, Melissa Drum, DDS, MS[b],
P.D. Eleazer, DDS, MS[c]

KEYWORDS

• Endodontic • Implant • Esthetic • Restoration

Dental professionals often face challenges when formulating a treatment plan for patients presenting with a compromised tooth, and have a duty to provide appropriate care for these patients to maintain dental health and esthetics. A common dilemma involves the decision between tooth retention using endodontic treatment with crown restoration, and extraction and an implant-borne restoration. Endodontic and implant restorations are performed daily by dentists and specialists. For endodontic treatment, estimates for the year 2000 were 30 million endodontic procedures annually (American Diabetes Association), while the number of patients receiving endosseous implants were estimated annually at 300,000 to 400,000 in 1996 and 910,000 in 2000 (Millennium Research Group). This may be a conservative estimate, according to the authors, because there has been an average growth rate increase of more than 40% annually for the 10-year period from 1997 to 2007 at the University of Minnesota (**Fig. 1**). In the year 2008, for the first time, the authors had seen a drop in the number of patients receiving implants, and this may have been because of the economic downturn or the generational changes that were occurring (in that the authors are now seeing less completely edentulous patients, while their partially edentulous patient population continues to increase).

OUTCOMES

In deciding on an appropriate treatment plan, the outcomes of treatment play a key role. The definition of success for dental implant studies is often implant survival, whereas root canal studies measure the healing of existing disease and the

This work was supported in part by a research grant from the American Association of Endodontists Foundation.
[a] Department of Restorative Sciences, University of Minnesota School of Dentistry, 515 Delaware Street SE, Minneapolis, MN 55455, USA
[b] Department of Endodontics, The Ohio State University School of Dentistry, 305 West 12th Avenue, PO Box 182357, Columbus, OH 43218, USA
[c] Department of Endodontics and Pulp Biology, University of Alabama at Birmingham, 4256 Sharpsburg Drive, Birmingham, AL 35213, USA
* Corresponding author.
E-mail address: bowle001@umn.edu

Dent Clin N Am 54 (2010) 401–413
doi:10.1016/j.cden.2009.12.008
0011-8532/10/$ – see front matter © 2010 Elsevier Inc. All rights reserved.

dental.theclinics.com

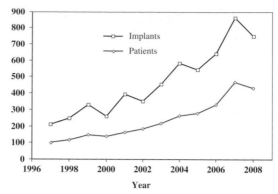

Fig. 1. Number of patients receiving implant treatment at the University of Minnesota and the total number of implants placed from 1997 to 2008.

occurrence of new disease.[1] The use of lenient success criteria in implant studies may translate to higher success rates, whereas stringent criteria used in root canal studies may lead to lower success rates.[2–4] To establish accurate comparisons, it is critical that the same outcome measures be used to assess endodontic and implant restorations. Because of these differences in the meanings of success, it is probable that survival rates will permit less biased, albeit less informative comparisons.[1,5–7] Often the stringent criteria in past endodontic studies have labeled some cases as failures when they were healing.[8]

Other factors can also affect outcomes, such as the restorative impact with endodontics. It has been shown that unrestored endodontically treated teeth were significantly more likely (4 times) to undergo extraction.[9] This restorative impact has been demonstrated by many investigators.[10–15] Examples of how restorations on endodontically treated and severely damaged teeth fail are shown in **Box 1**. Suggested restoration guidelines are shown in the flow chart shown in **Fig. 2**. Before using the flow chart, preliminary steps need to be done, which are shown in **Box 2**.

When evaluating the quality of the root canal treatment, common misconceptions surround what can or cannot be addressed with retreatments, endodontic surgery,

---

Box 1
How restorations on endodontically treated and severely damaged teeth fail

1. Stress breaks anatomic crown at the neck of the tooth

   a. Not strong enough ferrule (length and thickness)

   b. Core/tooth structure interface fails, shell of tooth structure suffers from stress, tooth structure fracture, crown fracture

Solution: Unless there is adequate length and thickness of ferrule, extract the tooth. Unless there is enough tooth structure available for mechanical retention or bonding, use cast dowel and core.

2. Cast dowel and core comes out from the root cement because it is not strong enough to withstand stress, especially under lateral or para-functional stress

Solution: Use resin cement for cast dowel and core and prefabricated post.

(*Courtesy of* Dr Wook-Jin Seong.)

and other treatments. Unfortunately, many of these teeth are deemed hopeless when that is not the case.

Fig. 2 can be used as a guideline to assist in treatment planning, although it may not fit every scenario precisely.

COSTS

In formulating patient treatment plans, costs often play an increasingly important role. Analysis of insurance data of 2005 concluded that restored single-tooth implants cost 75% to 90% more than similarly restored endodontic-treated teeth. Using mean United States fees, the implant restoration costs twice as much as endodontic restoration.[22] Examination of treatment costs at university settings have shown that implants cost more than twice as much (230%) as similar endodontically restored teeth (Bowles WR, Drum MM, Eleazer PE, unpublished data, 2009).[23] In addition, post-treatment complications are more common with implant restorations,[7,23–25] and these problems may increase this cost difference.

NEW STUDIES NEEDED

Patients prefer that their dentists use the best techniques and materials available. These advances in endodontics and implant treatment make some older studies less relevant. Because advanced materials and techniques come into use, success rates may be affected, which suggests the need for new outcome studies. For example, the use of intracanal medicaments in endodontics has changed over time.[26,27] Endodontic access openings are seldom left open, which allowed additional microbial contamination.[28,29] A retrospective look at endodontic surgery using newer techniques and instruments (no root-end bevel, ultrasonic instruments) found a twofold increase in success rate compared with older methods (91.1% vs 44.2%).[30] Endodontic treatment now includes the use of dental operating microscopes for better visibility, and hand instrumentation combined with nickel-titanium rotary instrumentation. Newer materials such as sustained-release antibacterial agents and new forms of mineral trioxide aggregate allow for potentially better treatment and call for additional outcome studies.

Advances in implants also continue to occur with improvements in such areas as shape, implant surface modifications, interface changes, and immediate placement. Previously, with implant placement 1.0 mm of bone loss during the first year of placement with an additional 0.1 mm annual loss was expected,[23,31,32] but this can vary with newer implant designs and materials. Although longevity outcomes for implant restorations are high, one recently reported concern is that patients with dental implant restorations have significantly lower maximum bite forces and reduced chewing efficiency compared with contralateral natural teeth, or even with endodontic restorations.[33]

Using matched implant and endodontic restorations in patients, the authors found similar longevity outcomes for endodontic and implant restorations (**Fig. 3**).

Several factors seem to be associated with higher failure rate of endodontic treatment. Smokers had an endodontic failure rate significantly (4 times) higher than nonsmokers (**Fig 4A**), whereas diabetic patients had almost a threefold increase in their failure rate (**Fig 4B**). Smoking and diabetes have previously been found to be a risk indicator for apical periodontitis.[34–36] In endodontic restorations, restoration with a post was also associated with a higher failure rate as seen in **Fig 5**. Earlier studies had suggested that the presence of posts do not affect the outcome of endodontic treatment.[37,38]

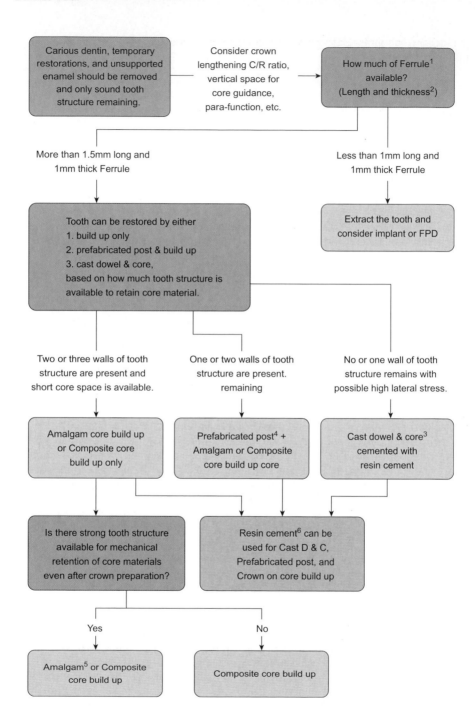

> **Box 2**
> **Preliminary steps to be done before using flow chart**
>
> 1. Complete evaluation of the whole mouth, in tandem with the particular tooth in question, so that a clear and comprehensive treatment plan can be formulated
>
> 2. Data collection
>
>   a. Periodontal support
>
>   b. Quality of root canal treatment
>
>   c. Occlusal scheme
>
>   d. Para-function
>
>   e. Intended tooth function: single restoration or abutment of fixed partial denture, removable partial denture, and overdenture
>
>   f. Vertical space available for the crown
>
> (*Courtesy of* Dr Wook-Jin Seong.)

Endo/Implant:Survival proportions

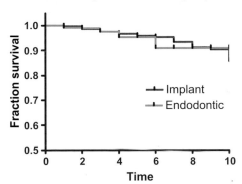

Fig 3. Survival proportions of implant and endodontic restorations. Outcome is not significantly different between groups (n = 4477).

Fig. 2. Restorations on endodontically treated and severely damaged teeth. Footnotes provide information for particular areas covered in this figure, and are described as follows. [1]Libman and Nicolls[16] found that crown preparation designs tested with lateral cyclic stress with ferrule of length 0.5 to 1.0 mm failed at a significantly lower number of cycles than ferrule length of 1.5 to 2.0 mm . [2]Pilo and colleagues[17] found that all the fractures occurred in the tooth structure and not in core materials. [3]Creugers and colleagues[18] conducted meta-analysis and reported 81% survival rate for composite cores with screw prefabricated post and 91% for cast dowel and cores for 6 years. [4]Tjan and colleagues[19] found amalgam core retained by a post was significantly stronger than amalgam cores retained by slots or channels. [5]Kovarik and colleagues[20] showed significant differences in the fatigue failure tests, with glass ionomer core experiencing total failure of all crowns by taking 20,000 cycles, composite core experiencing 80% failure by 50,000 cycles, and amalgam core experiencing 30% failure by 70,000 cycles. [6]Howdle and colleagues[21] found that adhesive resin luting cement significantly decreases the microleakage around crown margins where core restorations of amalgam or composite have been used. (*Courtesy of* Dr Wook-Jin Seong.)

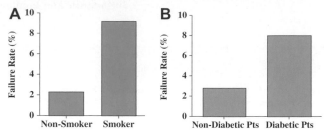

Fig. 4. (*A*) Failure rate for endodontic treatment in patients who smoke (*P* = .0013). (*B*) Failure rate for endodontic treatment in patients with diabetes.

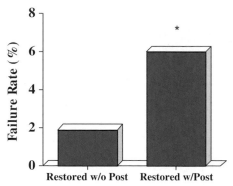

Fig. 5. Failure rate in endodontic restorations associated with posts (*P* = .0015).

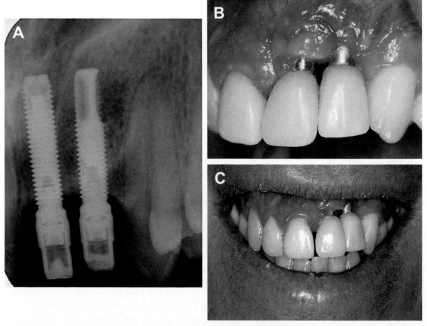

Fig. 6. Although the implants in (*A*) appear osseointegrated, the esthetic results are less than desirable (*B*, *C*). (*Courtesy of* Dr Deborah Johnson.)

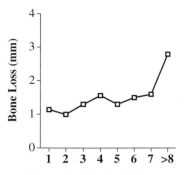

Years after Implant Placememt

Fig. 7. Mean crestal bone loss around implants.

Outcomes for implant restorations can also be affected by several factors. Care must be taken to preserve the esthetics with anterior implants, while obtaining osseointegration of the implant (**Fig. 6**). In earlier-implant patients, crestal bone loss occurred over the years; however, many newer implants may have decreased loss in the crestal bone. The authors have graphically presented the bone loss around implants over time (**Fig. 7**) for patients in their current study. Significant bone loss can be observed in younger patients receiving implant treatment by the time they reach old age.

In the authors' current study, implant restorations were less successful with diabetic patients, but did not seem to be affected by smoking, contrary to current literature results.[23,39,40] Implant restorations in diabetic patients had a 7.2% failure rate, compared with a failure rate of 4.1% in nondiabetic patients (**Fig. 8A**). Current literature suggests a 9% implant loss rate with controlled diabetes.[23,41–44] There was no significant difference in failure rates with implant restorations in patients who smoked compared with those who did not smoke (**Fig. 8B**).

For both types of treatment, gender or ethnicity has had no effect on outcome success. Also, the location of the endodontic treatment or implant placement did not significantly affect outcome.

To provide appropriate care, treatment must be preformed at a high-quality skill level for complex cases. Initial radiographs before starting endodontic treatment,

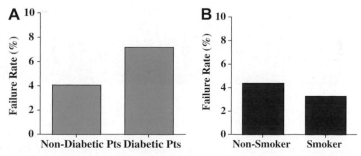

Fig. 8. (*A*) Failure rates of implant restorations in diabetic patients. (*B*) Failure rates of implant restorations in patients who smoke.

being only 2-dimensional, may not show the complexities associated with the pulp canal system (**Fig. 9**).

NEW TECHNOLOGY

Newer instruments and technology may be beneficial to endodontic and implant treatment modalities. Improvements in radiography have changed the algorithm of treatment. Endodontic cases can now use cone beam computed tomography (CT) scans for the evaluation of bone destruction caused by periapical lesions (**Fig. 10**).

Cone beam CT may also be used to improve diagnosis and treatment in implant placement whereby esthetics may be compromised. In **Fig. 11**, a fracture in the tooth led to loss of labial bone, which could not be detected clinically. By use of this advance in radiography, the treating practitioner is better informed and able to provide proper care for the patient while placing an immediate implant with bone graft.

Use of cone beam CT for better anatomic placement of implants and prevention of problems such as nerve injury are also becoming more frequent. Altered sensation after mandibular implant placement can result from trauma to any of the branches of the mandibular nerve.[45] With mental nerve neuropathy cases, invasive

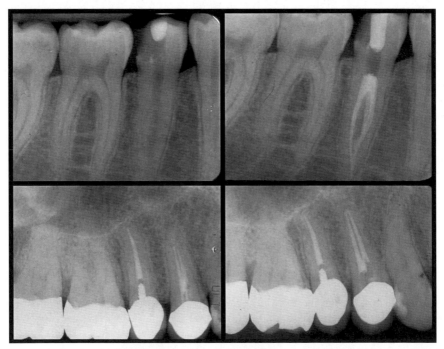

Fig. 9. Endodontic initial radiographs do not always show the complexities associated with canal systems. In **Fig 2**A, the mandibular second premolar has 3 canals, which can be difficult to obturate as shown in **Fig 2**B. In **Fig 2**C, a radiograph from a patient presenting with swelling around the periradicular area of tooth #5 shows inadequate instrumentation and obturation, to which the practitioner suggested implants for #4 and #5. Subsequent endodontic retreatment by a different practitioner was completed with successful results, and a recall radiograph is shown in **Fig 2**D. (*Courtesy of* Dr James Wolcott.)

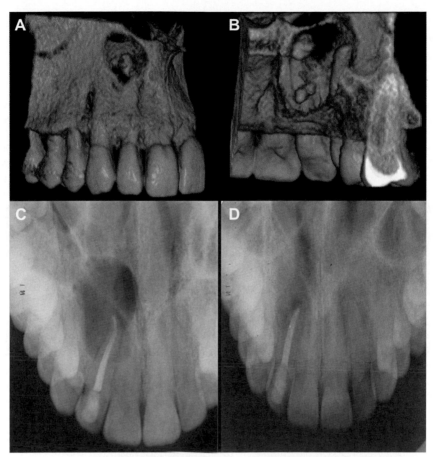

Fig 10. Periradicular lesion size can be large in presenting patients. Cone beam CT 3-dimensional reconstruction of periradicular lesion facial (*A*) and lingual (*B*). (*C*) A preoperative radiograph. (*D*) A recall radiograph after conventional and surgical retreatment. (*Courtesy of* Dr Joseph Petrino and Dr Mansur Ahmad.)

dental procedures (extractions, implants) were the etiologic factors in 63% of the cases.[46] The close proximity of the inferior alveolar nerve to tooth apices and possible implants placed in these extraction sites of mandibular posterior teeth are shown in **Fig. 12**.

Research is needed regarding immediate loading and compromised bone conditions (trauma, infection, systemic disease).[47] Also needed are improvements in bioactivity of dental implants to allow recruitment of osteoblasts, periodontal biosealing, and antimicrobial release.[48] Implant stability measurement by resonance frequency analysis may help evaluate osseointegration quickly and efficiently. [49,50]

SUMMARY

Functional survival rates are high for implant and endodontic restorations; however, areas for improvement exist for both treatment modalities. Related areas of implants

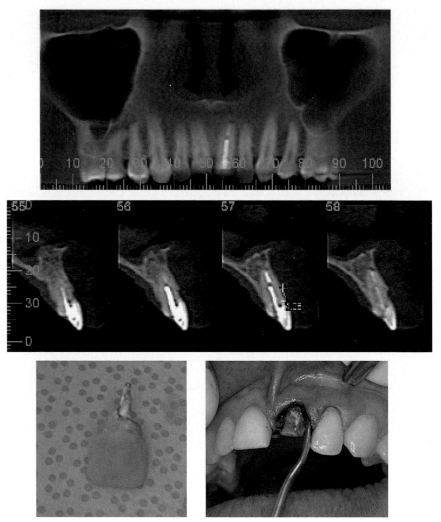

Fig. 11. Loss of labial bone was detected from fractured root of central incisor. (*Courtesy of James E. Hinrichs, DDS, MS and Mansur Ahmad, DDS, PhD.*)

include implant delivered pharmacology, faster integration, and decreased crestal bone loss, whereas related areas of endodontics include better seal (coronal and apical), improved disinfection of the pulp canal system (which suggests a role for antimicrobials such as 3MP [macrogol mixed with propylene glycol] paste[51] as intracanal medicaments), and better anatomic diagnosis (use of clinical micro-CT for 3-dimensional visualization of tooth with minimal radiation).

Endodontic treatment should be given priority in the treatment planning for periodontally sound teeth with pulpal or periradicular pathology, whereas implants should be given priority in the treatment planning for teeth that are to be extracted because of nonrestorability or other reasons. The decision between retention and extraction of a compromised tooth involves many factors that may influence the outcome, with

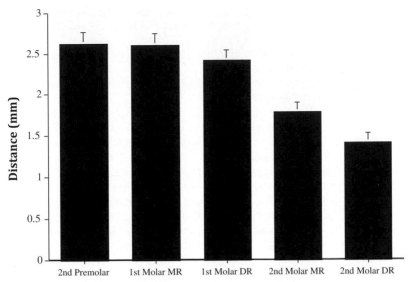

Fig. 12. Distance from mandibular tooth apices to inferior alveolar canal. Data were obtained through cone beam CT scans of randomly selected patients. Tooth apices of the mesial and distal roots of the second molar were significantly closer to the nerve (*P*<.001). (*Courtesy of* Tyler Koivisto and Dr Walter Bowles.)

the evaluation of restorability being critical. Because outcomes are similar with both treatments, decisions should be based on the patient's informed decision concerning restorability, costs associated with the procedures, esthetics, potential adverse outcomes, and ethical factors.

REFERENCES

1. Torabinejad M, Anderson P, Bader J, et al. Outcomes of root canal treatment and restoration, implant-supported single crowns, fixed partial dentures, and extraction without replacement: a systematic review. J Prosthet Dent 2007;98(4): 285–311.
2. Watson CJ, Tinsley D, Ogden AR, et al. A 3 to 4 year study of single tooth hydroxylapatite coated endosseous dental implants. Braz Dent J 1999;187(2):90–4.
3. Johnson RH, Persson GR. A 3-year prospective study of a single-tooth implant—prosthodontic complications. Int J Prosthodont 2001;14(2):183–9.
4. Wennström JL, Ekestubbe A, Gröndahl K, et al. Implant-supported single-tooth restorations: a 5-year prospective study. J Clin Periodontol 2005;32(6): 567–74.
5. Eckert SE, Wollan PC. Retrospective review of 1170 endosseous implants placed in partially edentulous jaws. J Prosthet Dent 1998;79(4):415–21.
6. Creugers NH, Kreulen CM, Snoek PA, et al. A systematic review of single-tooth restorations supported by implants. J Dent 2000;28(4):209–17.
7. Doyle SL, Hodges JS, Pesun IJ, et al. Retrospective cross sectional comparison of initial nonsurgical endodontic treatment and single-tooth implants. J Endod 2006;32(9):822–7.
8. Strindberg LZ. The dependence of the results of pulp therapy on certain factors. Acta Odontol Scand 1956;14(Suppl 21):1–179.

9. Lazarski MP, Walker WA 3rd, Flores CM, et al. Epidemiological evaluation of the outcomes of nonsurgical root canal treatment in a large cohort of insured dental patients. J Endod 2001;27(12):791–6.

10. Sorensen JA, Martinoff JT. Endodontically treated teeth as abutments. J Prosthet Dent 1985;53(5):631–6.

11. Vire DE. Failure of endodontically treated teeth: classification and evaluation. J Endod 1991;17(7):338–42.

12. Fraga RC, Chaves BT, Mello GS, et al. Fracture resistance of endodontically treated roots after restoration. J Oral Rehabil 1998;25(11):809–13.

13. Hoen MM, Pink FE. Contemporary endodontic retreatments: an analysis based on clinical treatment findings. J Endod 2002;28(12):834–6.

14. Aquilino SA, Caplan DJ. Relationship between crown placement and the survival of endodontically treated teeth. J Prosthet Dent 2002;87(3):256–63.

15. Salehrabi R, Rotstein I. Endodontic treatment outcomes in a large patient population in the USA: an epidemiological study. J Endod 2004;30(12):846–50.

16. Libman WJ, Nicholls JI. Load fatigue of teeth restored with cast posts and cores and complete crowns. Int J Prosthodont 1995;8(2):155–61.

17. Pilo R, Cardash HS, Levin E, et al. Effect of core stiffness on the in vitro fracture of crowned, endodontically treated teeth. J Prosthet Dent 2002;88(3):302–6.

18. Creugers NH, Mentink AG, Käyser AF. An analysis of durability data on post and core restorations. J Dent 1993;21(5):281–4.

19. Tjan AH, Dunn JR, Lee JK. Fracture resistance of amalgam and composite resin cores retained by various intradentinal retentive features. Quintessence Int 1993; 24(3):211–7.

20. Kovarik RE, Breeding LC, Caughman WF. Fatigue life of three core materials under simulated chewing conditions. J Prosthet Dent 1992;68(4):584–90.

21. Howdle MD, Fox K, Youngson CC. An in vitro study of coronal microleakage around bonded amalgam coronal-radicular cores in endodontically treated molar teeth. Quintessence Int 2002;33(1):22–9.

22. Christensen GJ. Implant therapy versus endodontic therapy. J Am Dent Assoc 2006;137(10):1440–3.

23. Goodacre CJ, Bernal G, Rungcharassaeng K, et al. Clinical complications with implants and implant prostheses. J Prosthet Dent 2003;90(2):121–32.

24. Iqbal MK, Kim S. For teeth requiring endodontic treatment, what are the differences in outcomes of restored endodontically treated teeth compared to implant-supported restorations? Int J Oral Maxillofac Implants 2007;(22 Suppl):96–116.

25. Hannahan JP, Eleazer PD. Comparison of success of implants versus endodontically treated teeth. J Endod 2008;34(11):1302–5.

26. Hasselgren G, Reit C. Emergency pulpotomy: pain relieving effect with and without the use of sedative dressings. J Epilepsy 1989;15(6):254–6.

27. Walton RE. Intracanal medicaments. Dent Clin North Am 1984;28(4):783–96.

28. Siqueira JF Jr. Microbial causes of endodontic flare-ups. Int Endod J 2003;36(7): 453–63.

29. Bence R, Meyers RD, Knoff RV. Evaluation of 5000 endodontic treatments: incidence of the opened tooth. Oral Surg Oral Med Oral Pathol 1980;49(1):82–4.

30. Tsesis I, Rosen E, Schwartz-Arad D, et al. Retrospective evaluation of surgical endodontic treatment: traditional versus modern technique. J Endod 2006; 32(5):412–6.

31. Henry PJ, Tolman DE, Bolender C. The applicability of osseointegrated implants in the treatment of partially edentulous patients: three-year results of a prospective multicenter study. Quintessence Int 1993;24(2):123–9.

32. Andersson B, Odman P, Lindvall AM, et al. Single-tooth restorations supported by osseointegrated implants: results and experiences from a prospective study after 2 to 3 years. Int J Oral Maxillofac Implants 1995;10(6):702–11.

33. Woodmansey KF, Ayik M, Buschang PH, et al. Differences in masticatory function in patients with endodontically treated teeth and single-implant-supported prostheses: a pilot study. J Endod 2009;35(1):10–4.

34. Kirkevang LL, Wenzel A. Risk indicators for apical periodontitis. Community Dent Oral Epidemiol 2003;31(1):59–67.

35. Fouad AF. Diabetes mellitus as a modulating factor of endodontic infections. J Dent Educ 2003;67(4):459–67.

36. Fouad AF, Burleson J. The effect of diabetes mellitus on endodontic treatment outcome: data from an electronic patient record. J Am Dent Assoc 2003; 134(1):43–51.

37. Tronstad L, Asbjørnsen K, Døving L, et al. Influence of coronal restorations on the periapical health of endodontically treated teeth. Endod Dent Traumatol 2000; 16(5):218–21.

38. Friedman S, Abitbol S, Lawrence HP. Treatment outcome in endodontics: the Toronto Study. Phase 1: initial treatment. J Endod 2003;29(12):787–93.

39. Bain CA, Moy PK. The association between the failure of dental implants and cigarette smoking. Int J Oral Maxillofac Implants 1993;8(6):609–15.

40. Wallace RH. The relationship between cigarette smoking and dental implant failure. Eur J Prosthodont Restor Dent 2000;8(3):103–6.

41. Balshi SF, Wolfinger GJ, Balshi TJ. An examination of immediately loaded dental implant stability in the diabetic patient using resonance frequency analysis (RFA). Quintessence Int 2007;38(4):271–9.

42. Fiorellini JP, Chen PK, Nevins M, et al. A retrospective study of dental implants in diabetic patients. Int J Periodontics Restorative Dent 2000;20(4):366–73.

43. Olson JW, Shernoff AF, Tarlow JL, et al. Dental endosseous implant assessments in a type 2 diabetic population: a prospective study. Int J Oral Maxillofac Implants 2000;15(6):811–8.

44. Morris HF, Ochi S, Winkler S. Implant survival in patients with type 2 diabetes: placement to 36 months. Ann Periodontol 2000;5(1):157–65.

45. Kraut RA, Chahal O. Management of patients with trigeminal nerve injuries after mandibular implant placement. J Am Dent Assoc 2002;133(10):1351–4.

46. Kalladka M, Proter N, Benoliel R, et al. Mental nerve neuropathy: patient characteristics and neurosensory changes. Oral Surg Oral Med Oral Pathol Oral Radiol Endod 2008;106(3):364–70.

47. Schliephake H, Aref A, Scharnweber D, et al. Effect of modifications of dual acid-etched implant surfaces on peri-implant bone formation. Part I: organic coatings. J Clin Oral Implants Res 2009;20(1):31–7.

48. Manero JM, Salsench J, Nogueras J, et al. Growth of bioactive surfaces on dental implants. Implant Dent 2002;11(2):170–5.

49. Meredith N. Assessment of implant stability as a prognostic determinant. Int J Prosthodont 1998;11(5):491–501.

50. Sennerby L, Meredith N. Implant stability measurements using resonance frequency analysis: biological and biomechanical aspects and clinical implications. Periodontol 2000 2008;47:51–66.

51. Takushige T, Cruz EV, Asgor Moral A, et al. Endodontic treatment of primary teeth using a combination of antibacterial drugs. Int Endod J 2004;37(2):132–8.

Index

Note: Page numbers of article titles are in **boldface** type.

Dent Clin N Am 54 (2010) 415–422
doi:10.1016/S0011-8532(10)00013-3
0011-8532/10/$ – see front matter © 2010 Elsevier Inc. All rights reserved.

dental.theclinics.com

Moving?

Make sure your subscription moves with you!

To notify us of your new address, find your **Clinics Account Number** (located on your mailing label above your name), and contact customer service at:

Email: journalscustomerservice-usa@elsevier.com

800-654-2452 (subscribers in the U.S. & Canada)
314-447-8871 (subscribers outside of the U.S. & Canada)

Fax number: 314-447-8029

Elsevier Health Sciences Division
Subscription Customer Service
3251 Riverport Lane
Maryland Heights, MO 63043